Systemic Anti-Cancer Therapy for Nurses

This text introduces and explains all aspects of systemic anti-cancer therapy, from pharmacology to administration and beyond, providing the underpinning knowledge to support completion of the UKONS SACT competency passport.

Written by experienced practitioners and lecturers, this concise book:

- critically analyses how the pharmacological properties of anti-cancer drugs and their role at various stages of the cell cycle impacts on their administration;
- examines the management of patients receiving systemic anti-cancer therapy;
- explores the health and safety, professional and legal aspects of administration of anti-cancer drug therapy;
- appraises the holistic needs of patients receiving systemic anti-cancer therapy.

Each chapter includes case scenarios, illustrations, further reading and self-assessment exercises to aid learning.

This is the perfect book for nurses who are undertaking a university-accredited systemic anti-cancer therapy course or are new to practising in the field.

Alison Simons is a Senior Lecturer in Cancer at Birmingham City University with 18 years' experience as a cancer nurse in a teaching hospital, including leadership of an oncology ward and staff development.

Samantha Toland is a Nurse Consultant and Lead SACT nurse with 26 years in clinical practice within oncology/haemato-oncology.

Emma Filby is a Senior Lecturer and Course Lead in Applied Cancer Practice at Birmingham City University, and an experienced senior cancer nurse with over 15 years' experience in cancer services.

Systemic Anti-Cancer Therapy for Nurses

A Guide to Principles, Practice and Care

Alison Simons, Samantha Toland and Emma Filby

Routledge
Taylor & Francis Group
LONDON AND NEW YORK

Designed cover image: Getty Images

First published 2027
by Routledge
4 Park Square, Milton Park, Abingdon, Oxon OX14 4RN

and by Routledge
605 Third Avenue, New York, NY 10158

Routledge is an imprint of the Taylor & Francis Group, an informa business

British Library Cataloguing-in-Publication Data
A catalogue record for this book is available from the British Library

Library of Congress Cataloging-in-Publication Data
Names: Simons, Alison author | Toland, Samantha author | Filby, Emma author
Title: Systematic anti-cancer therapy for nurses : a guide to principles, practice and care / Alison Simons, Samantha Toland, Emma Filby.
Description: Abingdon, Oxon ; New York, NY : Routledge, 2026. |
Includes bibliographical references and index.
Identifiers: LCCN 2026023550 (print) | LCCN 2026023551 (ebook) |
ISBN 9781032850856 hbk | ISBN 9781032850788 pbk | ISBN 9781003516477 ebk
Subjects: LCSH: Cancer–Nursing
Classification: LCC RC266 .S47 2026 (print) | LCC RC266 (ebook)
LC record available at https://lccn.loc.gov/2026023550
LC ebook record available at https://lccn.loc.gov/2026023551

ISBN: 978-1-032-85085-6 (hbk)
ISBN: 978-1-032-85078-8 (pbk)
ISBN: 978-1-003-51647-7 (ebk)

DOI: 10.4324/9781003516477

Typeset in Sabon
by Newgen Publishing UK

Contents

About the Authors

Alison Simons is a Senior Lecturer in cancer with 18 years' experience as a cancer nurse in a teaching hospital, including leadership of an oncology ward and staff development. Passionate about nurse education, she has led education, induction and competency development across oncology and haematology services. Alison joined Birmingham City University in 2009 and leads modules within the Applied Cancer Practice Course. Her research focuses on chemotherapy safety, with publications, presentations and European policy work.

Samantha Toland is an experienced cancer and haemato-oncology nurse with 26 years in clinical practice. Her roles have included stem cell transplant nursing, chemotherapy nurse trainer, leukaemia nurse specialist, acute oncology nurse practitioner and lead chemotherapy nurse across a multi-site trust. Sam held an academic post at Birmingham City University and published on hazardous drug safety. She is now a Nurse Consultant in Cancer Care and Lead SACT Nurse, with national and regional leadership responsibilities.

Emma Filby is a Senior Lecturer and Course Lead in Applied Cancer Practice at Birmingham City University, and an experienced senior cancer nurse with over 15 years' experience in cancer services. She has led chemotherapy, acute oncology and specialist cancer nursing services across NHS organisations. Her clinical expertise includes systemic anti-cancer therapy, service development, governance and patient safety, alongside advancing practice-based cancer nursing education and workforce capability, and delivering safe, compassionate, evidence-based care in practice.

CHAPTER 1

Cell Biology

Alison Simons

Introduction

To understand how cancer is initiated and apply the mechanism of action of anti-cancer drugs, you first need to be able to understand normal cell biology and the cell cycle. The majority of this chapter will explore the normal cell, normal cell division, the cell cycle, and control of normal cell growth and division. As cancer is caused by unregulated cell growth and tumours are a group of mutated cells, the final part of this chapter will look at what happens when this regulated cell growth becomes unregulated and leads to the development of cancer.

The Cell – DNA, Genes, Chromosomes and Codons

Cells are the building blocks of the body, which are controlled by the nucleus. The nucleus contains the instructions the cell needs to replicate. The chromosomes within the nucleus are supercoiled structures of deoxyribonucleic acid (DNA) that are only visible when the cell is dividing. There are 46 chromosomes in human cells made up of 23 homologous pairs, numbered 1–22 and sex chromosomes X and Y (see Figure 1.1).

DNA is a double helix structure, which has 4 nucleotide bases: adenine (A), thymine (T), guanine (G) and cytosine (C) that make up each single strand. These bases pair up with the corresponding bases in the second strand like rungs of a ladder. Adenine will always pair with thymine, and guanine and cytosine will always pair together (Blows, 2025, pg 3) (see Figure 1.2).

Genes are a section of DNA that code for proteins. You could think of a gene as a recipe to make a protein. Proteins are made up of chains of amino acids; these are called polypeptide chains, some are made up of several chains of amino acids (multimeric proteins) such as haemoglobin, while others are made up of just one chain, such as insulin. The different structure of these chain(s) mean they twist and fold into 3D shapes

DOI: 10.4324/9781003516477-1

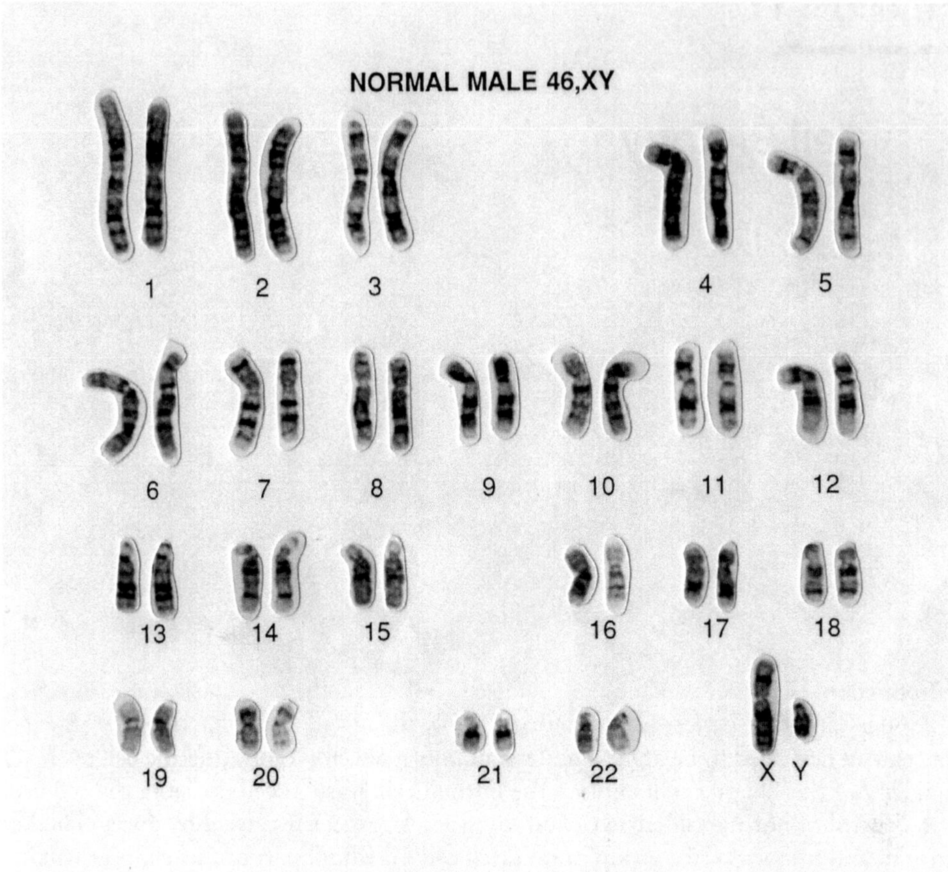

Figure 1.1 A typical human Karyotype

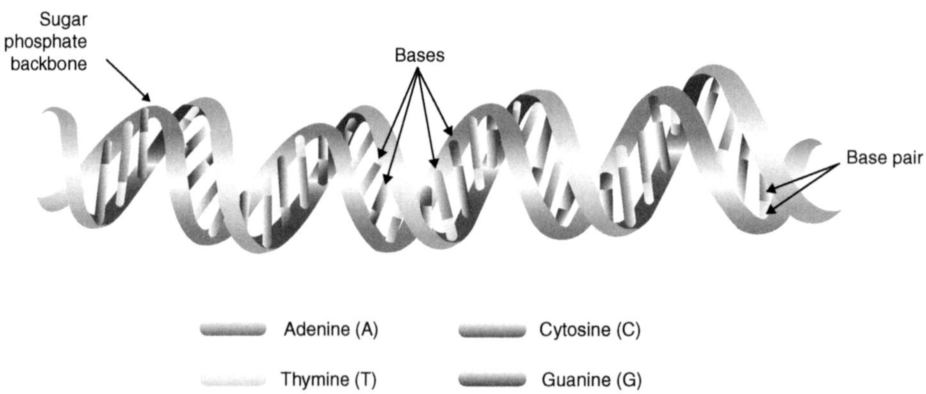

Figure 1.2 DNA double helix with nucleotide bases

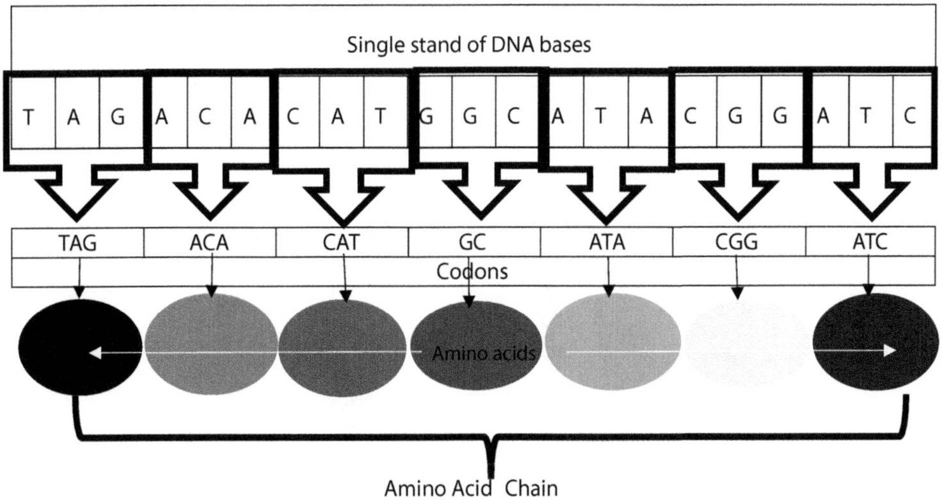

Figure 1.3 DNA, codons, amino acids and amino acid chain

which define the protein function. Each group of three DNA bases of the gene is called a codon (trinucleotide), and each codon codes for one amino acid (Vologodskii, 2023, pg 19). There are 20 known amino acids. The amino acids will be assembled in the same order that the codons appear in the gene's DNA strand. You could think of amino acids as the ingredients within the recipe to make a protein (See Figure 1.3).

Let's look at the process of how a protein is made from the recipe (Gene) and ingredients (amino acids). Firstly, the DNA double helix structure needs to be unravelled, and the two strands need to be separated so the recipe (genes and codons) can be read; a DNA polymerase (enzyme) facilitates this uncoiling of the DNA. When the long strands of DNA are unravelled (imagine this as an unravelled ball of wool) it is at risk of tangling or knotting. This makes reading the DNA bases very difficult and could risk damage or errors forming within the DNA strand. If you think about a very tangled and knotted ball of wool, sometimes the only way to release the wool would be to use scissors to cut a strand of wool to release the knot. Within DNA it is a similar process; to prevent or release this tangling and knotting of the DNA strand, an enzyme called topoisomerase II causes the DNA strands to be cut, allowing the tangle to be released. Topoisomerase II then reseals the DNA strands to prevent any further errors or tangling of the DNA strand. Once the DNA has been untangled it needs to be separated into two separate base strands so the genes can be read. An enzyme called helicase facilitates this by severing the hydrogen bonds that hold the two strands together. You could think of this like a stringy cheese stick being peeled apart. Now the single base strands are separated, the gene can now be read. The gene is transcribed into messenger ribonucleic acid (mRNA) by the enzyme RNA polymerase II. This mRNA is a complimentary copy of that gene (section of DNA) which then attaches to a ribosome, an organelle within the cell cytoplasm that can synthesise proteins that translates the RNA into amino acids (Vologodskii, 2023, pg 21). The ribosome reads the mRNA and assembles the correct amino acids in the correct sequence as instructed by the codons within the mRNA to form the protein chain (see Figure 1.4).

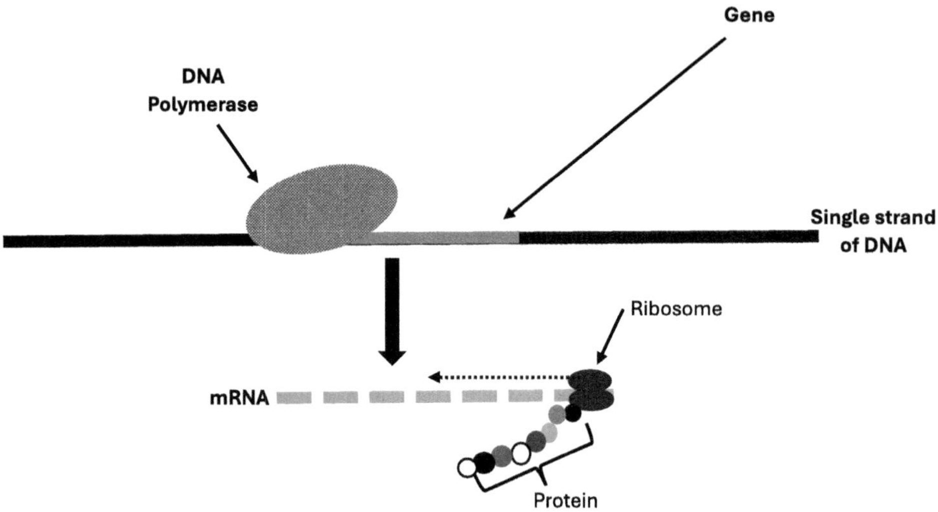

Figure 1.4 Protein transcription

Another way you could look at the cell is to think of it as a library, and within this library is a very special book (the nucleus). The 46 pages of the book are the chromosomes, genes are the sentences on the pages, codons and amino acids are the words, and the DNA bases are the letters of the words. Using this analogy, if for whatever reason something went wrong and the letters of the words in this book were misprinted or missing, it would alter the whole story of the book. This is the same within the cell; if something goes wrong with the DNA bases, the codons and thus the amino acids would not be in the correct order, meaning the gene would be in an incorrect order (potentially mutated). The incorrectly ordered (mutated) gene will code for a mutated protein which will have a detrimental effect. This will be particularly important to remember when we discuss genes that control cell growth later in the chapter.

Stop and Think ...

Can you explain each of these terms?

- Nucleus
- Chromosome
- Deoxyribose nucleic acid
- Nucleotide bases
- Gene
- Codon
- Amino acid

Cell Division

Most cells have the amazing ability to replicate themselves whenever it's required, through the process of cell division (a cyclical process). Cells that have been through cell division many times mean their DNA has been uncoiled, snipped, copied, resealed and recoiled several times over. This leads to a loss in elasticity of the DNA strand, and the DNA double helix structure in effect becomes 'baggy' and unstable as it does not coil back as tightly, and this increases the risk of DNA damage and inability to repair this damage. As the DNA has been copied several times there is also the risk of mutations, you could think of this as photocopying a copy of a copy of a copy of a document where the copied document is of poorer quality than the original document. This ultimately heightens the risk of DNA mutation and therefore induces apoptosis; in other words, the cell receives a message to say it is too damaged or at risk of developing mutations that it must commit cell suicide. This is an inbuilt anti-cancer mechanism within cells to minimise the risk of developing DNA and cellular mutations and destroying cells that have developed these mutations.

Once the apoptosis process starts, it triggers chemical messages to tell other cells to grow and divide because that cell needs to be replaced. You could think of this as if you have eaten a packet of salt and vinegar crisps. The mechanical action of eating these hard crisps, coupled with the acidic flavours cause the cells within your mouth to become damaged or destroyed. This induces repairs to your cell's damaged DNA or apoptosis. This triggers messages to be sent to your other mucosal membrane cells to tell

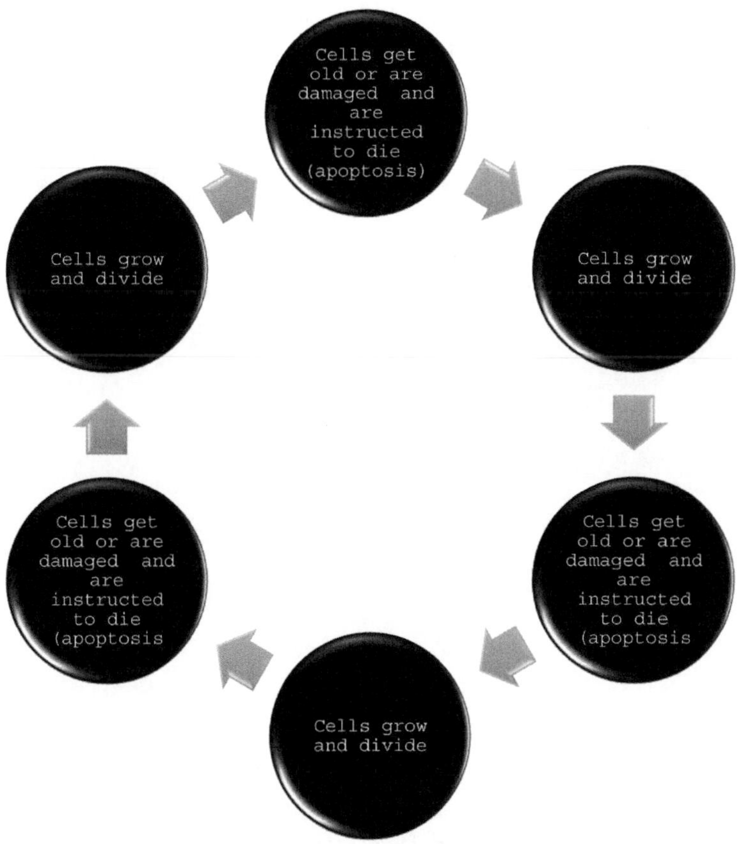

Figure 1.5 A basic overview of the sequence of cell replication

them they need to divide to replace your lost mucosal cells. So, it stimulates other cells to go through the cell cycle and divide. Once these cells get older or are damaged beyond repair they get instructed to die, which then triggers off a message for other cells to grow and so on. This means there are constantly exactly the right number of cells at any one time, never too many and never too few, and this is because of this tightly controlled cell division and cell growth (Figure 1.5).

Cell division is imperative because even the act of breathing means lung cells will constantly need replacing (Rote, 2019, pg 35). The complex and controlled process of cell division is happening all the time and usually without any issues; we will take a look at this in more detail later in the chapter and explore what happens when control of cell growth is lost.

Control of Cell Growth, Division and the Cell Cycle

Cell growth is a very complex and uniform process. On a basic level it is controlled by genes and growth factors. Previously in this chapter we talked about how genes code for proteins. The main genes involved in control of the cell cycle are proto-oncogenes and tumour suppressor genes (TSG). Proto-oncogenes code for proteins that promote cell growth, while TSG code for proteins that control the cell cycle by making DNA repairs or instruct apoptosis (cell death). You could think about this like driving a car. The proto-oncogene acts as the accelerator pedal while the TSG acts as the brake pedal. These genes are activated at the checkpoints within the cell cycle, and this will be illustrated in the cell cycle section in this chapter.

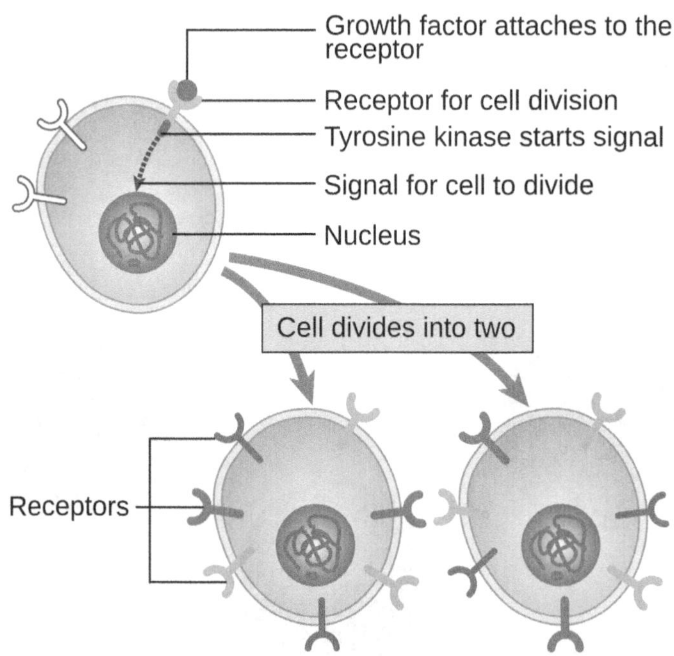

Figure 1.6 Diagram showing how growth factors signal to the cell to grow and divide

Growth factors (see Chapter 9) control cell division in a very targeted way; cells have many different growth factor receptors on their surface. Each receptor is very specific to certain cell line growth, for example, white blood cells, red blood cells, and blood vessels. Once a specific growth factor for a particular cell line has been released into the bloodstream, they will seek out cells with their specific growth factor receptors on their surface. This works on a lock and key hypothesis, in that only the correct growth factor will fit into their respective growth factor receptor. When the growth factor attaches to its correct receptor it will stimulate a chain reaction. This starts by sending a chemical message using protein kinases such as tyrosine kinase to the nucleus, instructing cell division to commence, and the cell will enter the cell cycle (See Figure 1.6).

Stop and Think ...
What is the function of the proto-oncogene?
What are the functions of the TSG?
Can you think of any growth factors you may use in treatment of SACT side effects?

The Cell Cycle
When cell growth and division is required, cells must progress through the cell cycle, the process by which a single cell undergoes cell division and divides into two identical daughter cells (Blows, 2025, pg 6). The cell cycle is controlled by many genes and stimulated by growth factors, which will be discussed later in this chapter.

The cell cycle is made up of 5 phases. G0, G1, S G2 (interphase) and M (mitotic phase); let's look at each of these in turn.

The G0 phase (resting or quiescent phase) is when the cell is not actively dividing; this does not mean the cell is resting as it is carrying out its cellular function of whatever that cell is. In other words, the cell is functioning but not cycling. Cells in the G0 phase can be recruited into the G1 phase when cell growth is instructed.

The G1 phase is the first growth phase, and this is when the cell begins preparation for division. The cell is producing and gathering what is required for division, such as RNA and then checks that it has everything it needs to move into the S phase. This phase lasts between 12 and 14 hours. At the end of the G1 phase there is a cell cycle checkpoint/restriction point. This is where the cell cycle pauses and it cannot pass into the next phase of division until it undergoes a spot check. If the cell does not have everything that is required to divide, it will have to gather what it needs. I think of this restriction point like a parent at the front door checking their child has everything they need for the school day ahead. If they are not ready as they do not have everything, then they need to go back and get their PE kit, reading book, etc. before they are allowed to leave the house. Also, at this checkpoint/restriction point the TSG proteins check for any errors or damage, and if detected will attempt to repair it. If the damage cannot be repaired then TSG proteins trigger apoptosis. Once this restriction point has been passed then the cell is committed to cell division and cannot go back. In my analogy this is when the child has now set off for school and cannot return to the house.

The S phase is the synthesis phase. To enable a single cell with 23 pairs of chromosomes to divide into two identical daughter cells (each with 23 pairs of chromosomes), the DNA needs to double (to make the total of 46 pairs of chromosomes), therefore synthesis of

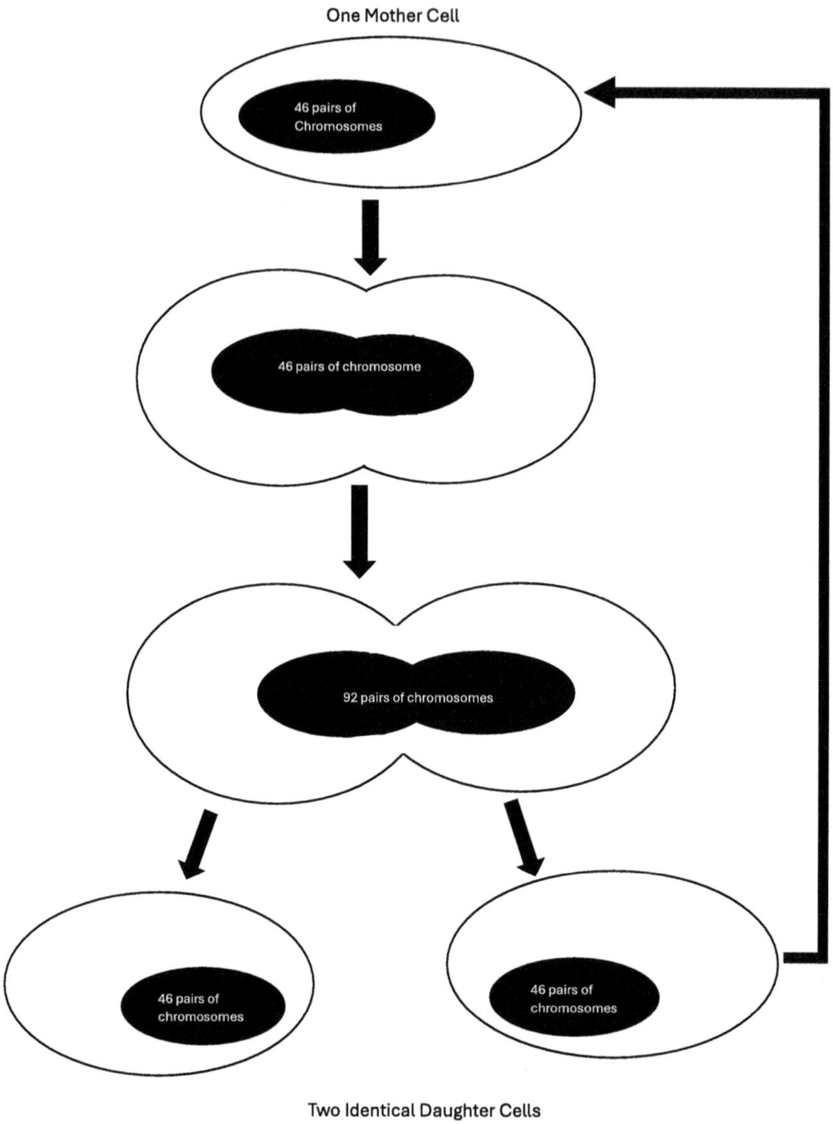

Figure 1.7 An overview of the process of cell division

DNA must be performed (see Figure 1.7). This phase lasts about 7–20 hours. This process begins with the uncoiling of the DNA double helix, an enzyme (DNA polymerase) untwists the DNA and the enzyme helicase allows the two nucleotide strands to peel away from each other (like the process we discussed in protein synthesis earlier in the chapter). Each single nucleotide strand then acts as a template for the construction of a complementary strand. So the result is that two DNA molecules are formed that are identical to the original DNA helix. Due to the process of uncoiling and separation of the DNA nucleotide chains, this is the phase when the cell is most vulnerable to damage or error (see Figure 1.8).

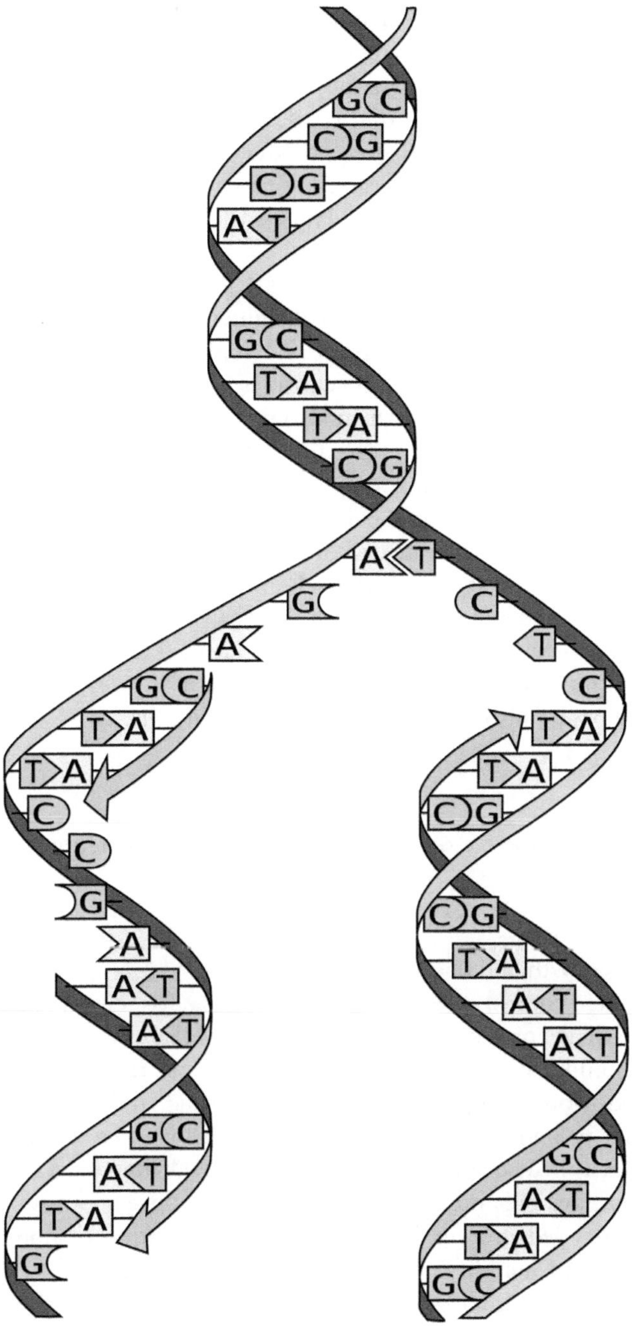

Figure 1.8 DNA synthesis

The G2 phase is the second growth and pre-mitotic phase and lasts 1–4 hours. In this phase synthesis of some additional proteins and RNA occurs. At the end of the G2 phase there is a second restriction point involving the TSG p53. The p53 gene is an important TSG as it codes for the p53 protein that regulates cell cycle progression and apoptosis. When DNA is damaged this leads to rapid production of p53, the cell cycle halts so the DNA can be repaired, or, if the DNA cannot be repaired then p53 is required to induce apoptosis, before replication to prevent damaged DNA being copied (Rote, 2019, pg 38) (see Figure 1.10).

M phase or mitotic phase lasts between 40 minutes and 2 hours and is when the mother cell physically splits into two daughter cells. It is made up of four sub phases: Prophase, Metaphase, Anaphase and Telophase (see Figure 1.9). Prophase is where the chromosomes condense, and centrioles moves to opposite poles of the cell. Metaphase involves the 46 pairs of chromosomes aligning across the cell equator. The nucleoli and nuclear membrane disappear during this sub phase, and spindles form from the centrioles across the cell. During anaphase the 46 chromosomes pairs separate into two identical sets of 23 chromosome pairs. One set is pulled to one end of the cell, and the other set is pulled to the opposite end of the cell, so there are two identical sets of 23 pairs of chromosomes at each end of the cell (Vologodskii, 2023, pg 47). Next within the telophase the chromosomes elongate, the nuclear membranes reappear and enclose around the chromosomes, and the centrioles replicate so there are two at each end of the cell. Finally, cytokinesis can occur where the cytoplasm divides, and the two daughter cells physically separate into two independent identical cells.

Stop and Think ...

Which phase of the cell cycle do you think is the most vulnerable to DNA damage? And why?

Unregulated Cell Growth and Cancer

The tightly regulated control of cell growth can go awry, for several reasons, for example acquired DNA damage or inherited genetic mutations (Saucedo and Jost, 2023, pg 79). Proto-oncogenes and TSG can become mutated and lose their ability to function correctly. A mutated proto-oncogene is called an oncogene, and this mutated gene codes for a protein that promotes cell growth; however, this is done in an unregulated way, resulting in uncontrolled cell growth and proliferation. A mutated TSG codes for a protein that does not have the ability to repair DNA and induce apoptosis in the same way as a normal TSG-coded protein. This results in proliferation of potentially damaged or mutated DNA and inability for these damaged or mutated cells to be destroyed. Thinking back to the car analogy, you could imagine that the oncogene is the accelerator pedal with a brick on it, so unable to stop the acceleration of the car. The mutated TSG could be a broken brake pedal, unable to slow down or stop the car. The result on a cellular level from either a mutated proto-oncogene (oncogene) and/or mutated TSG is the initiation and proliferation of mutated cells that are not able to be destroyed, in other words, a tumour.

Cancers are diseases that start with cells; tumours are a group of mutated cells. Oncology means the study of cells. The mutated cells that result from the unregulated

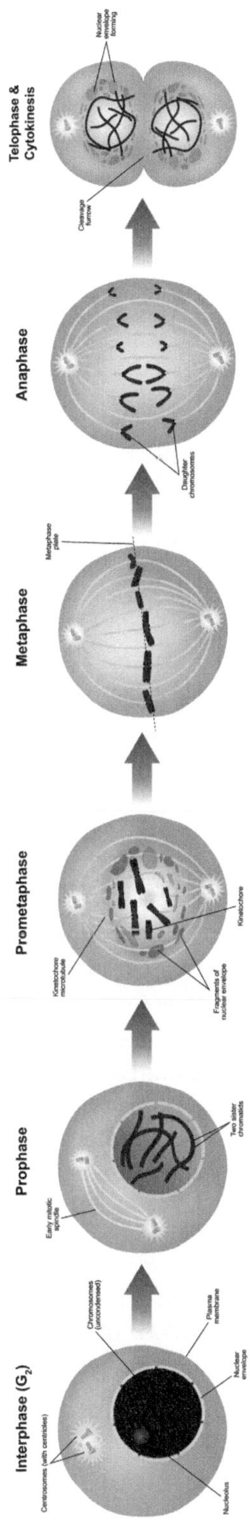

Figure 1.9 The stages of mitosis

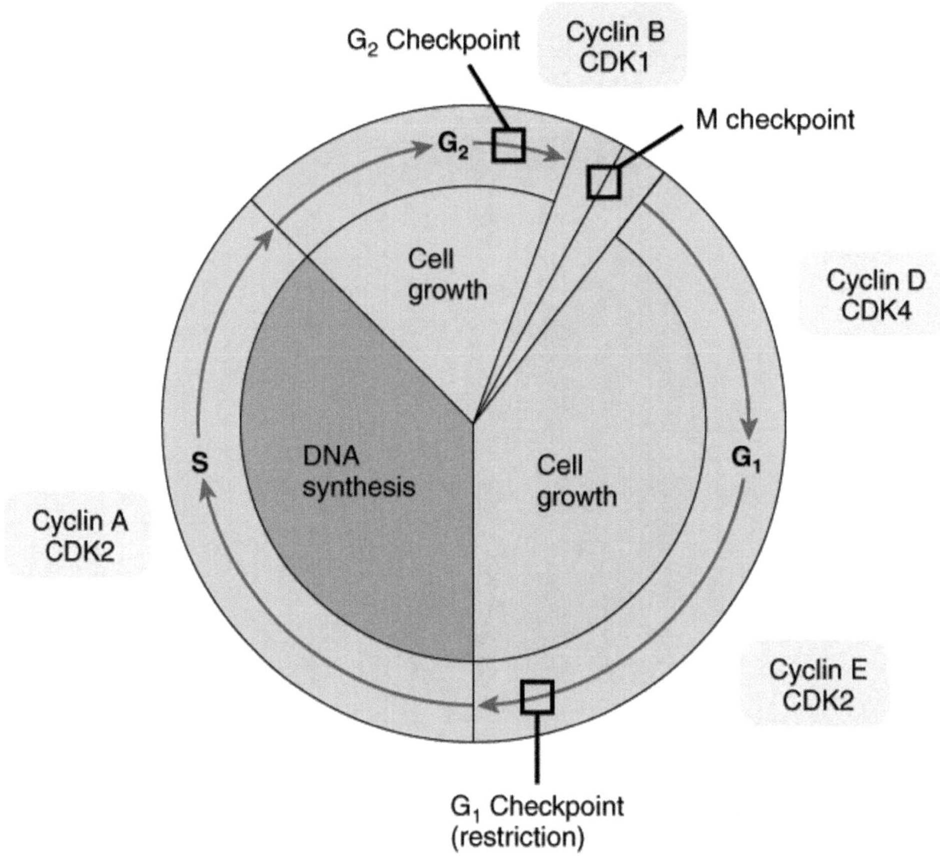

Figure 1.10 The phases of the cell cycle and checkpoints

cell growth can continue to undergo cell division and the cell cycle pretty much unnoticed. Remember we discussed earlier in the chapter that the TSG which would normally code for a protein to identify DNA damage and signal apoptosis (cell death) is not functioning correctly. Therefore, mutated cells continue to grow, divide and proliferate, invading into tissues and organs. If this unregulated cell growth is not identified and treated it can spread further into the whole system of the organ and eventually metastasise to other parts of the body such as the liver, lung and brain.

Summary

Cell growth, cell division, the cell cycle and cell death are carefully controlled, uniform and regulated by genes and growth factors. If one of these genes becomes damaged or mutated, then gene regulation will change and result in unregulated cell growth and tumour formation.

References

Blows, W.T. (2025) *The biological basis of cancer*. Second edition. Oxford: Routledge. doi:10.4324/9781003389125.

Rote, N.S. (2019) 'Chapter 12 – Cancer biology', in *Pathophysiology*. Eighth Edition [Online]. Elsevier Inc., Missouri, pp. 346–378.

Saucedo, L. and Jost, M. (2023) *Getting to know your cells*. 1st edition. Cham: Springer. doi:10.1007/978-3-031-30146-9.

Vologodskii, A. (2023) *The basics of molecular biology*. 1st edition. Cham: Springer. doi:10.1007/978-3-031-19404-7.

CHAPTER 2

Pharmacology of Anti-Cancer Drugs

Samantha Toland

Introduction

Many of the more traditional drugs that are used in the treatment of cancer are aimed at either directly killing cells (cytotoxic) or are used to prevent cell division (cytostatic). This is because the target of drug therapy is the differential between normal healthy cells and cancer cells – this being a more rapid rate of replication. Therefore, traditional chemotherapy agents mainly target cell DNA/replication. The origins of cytotoxic chemotherapy really date back to post second world war – where mustard gas had been used in warfare, it was noted that soldiers had bone marrow suppression as a result, hence the development of nitrogen mustard chemotherapy drugs, some of which are still used today (for example, Bendamustine).

Cell Fraction-Kill Hypothesis

Before we discuss the pharmacology of individual drugs, it is important to understand the principle of cell-kill hypothesis in cancer treatment. This is the theory that only a proportion of cancer cells will be killed with each cycle/round of treatment, requiring subsequent cycles of treatment to be administered. There are a number of reasons for this: firstly, the cancer may not be well supplied with blood in its entirety due to irregular angiogenesis (blood vessel development), therefore as the treatment is given systemically (via the blood stream) the treatment may not be able to reach parts of the cancer. Secondly, cancers can build resistance to drugs and therefore they may become less effective with time. Thirdly, not all cancer cells may be susceptible to death due to the stage of replication they are in (cells that are in G0 phase are less susceptible to the action of SACT). It is impossible to give treatment continuously due to the effects on normal healthy cells (these drugs do not differentiate between normal and cancerous cells) so we can only give treatments in bursts (usually known as a cycle) to allow cell recovery in between. This means that a number of cycles are usually required to enable

 DOI: 10.4324/9781003516477-2

the maximum cell-killing benefit. The rate of regrowth of cancers is also important as cancers can grow back during the recovery phase; hence the gaps between cycles are kept to a minimum which is generally 2–3 weeks (McFadden, 2019).

Cancer Response to Cytotoxic Chemotherapy

Different cancer types respond differently to cytotoxic drugs – this is due to the speed of proliferation of the cell of origin, so for example, haematological cancers generally respond well to cytotoxic chemotherapy as the cells of origin are blood cells which are already replicating rapidly. Slower growing cancers such as prostate cancers tend not to respond so well to cytotoxic treatment as the cell replication rate within prostate cancers is much slower.

Response to this type of treatment also depends on genetic factors – particularly cell cycle checkpoints (see Chapter 1); if there is a mutation present in particular genetic controls of the cell cycle, then a cell will not be recognised as damaged, and apoptosis (programmed cell death) will not automatically take place, affecting the impact of the chemotherapy treatment. A common genetic mutation occurs in the p53 gene which often results in a lack of response to cytotoxic chemotherapy.

Side Effects of Treatment

This will be discussed in Chapter 6, but fundamentally the range of side effects that are evident from traditional chemotherapy agents occurs due to the fact that they destroy any rapidly dividing cell types within the body – skin and hair cells, mucous membrane cells, bone marrow cells and germ cells (fertility) can all be destroyed by chemotherapy agents. This results in the unpleasant side effects that many patients experience – sore/ulcerated mouth, nausea/vomiting, diarrhoea/constipation, myelosuppression resulting in increased risk of infection, hair loss and infertility. Therefore, patients require time between cycles (usually 2–3 weeks) to allow cell recovery and enable them to have further treatment.

Pharmacology of Chemotherapy Agents

These agents can be separated into different groups according to their mechanism of action. They can be first separated into two categories: cell cycle phase specific, and cell cycle phase non-specific drugs. Chemotherapy agents can further be broken down into groups within these categories as outlined below.

Cell Cycle Phase Non-Specific Drugs

Cell cycle phase non-specific drugs are generally able to cause cell destruction regardless of which phase of replication the cell is in. So, a cell can be in G1 phase, it can be in S phase, it can be in G2, it can even be in mitosis and these drugs will have an impact. Some of these drugs can also work when the cell is in G0 phase (not replicating). These drugs are generally given as one-off doses as part of a treatment cycle as they tend to have a significant cell-killing effect on large numbers of cells in one go.

Alkylating Agents

This group of chemotherapy drugs work by creating cross-links between guanine bases within the DNA of cells (see Figure 2.1), thus rendering the cell incapable of replication, but also causing DNA mutation so that cell death (apoptosis) is induced (McFadden, 2019). Thus, these drugs will generally have an impact on DNA/cell replication regardless of which phase of replication the cell is in. Examples of these agents include cyclophosphamide, ifosphamide, bendamustine and the platinum agents – cisplatin, carboplatin and oxaliplatin. They are used in a wide range of cancers, but particularly haematological cancers (lymphomas and leukaemias) and the platinum agents are predominantly used in upper GI, lower GI, gynaecological and lung cancers.

Figure 2.1 shows a strand of DNA with its constituent base pairs – where there are two guanine bases in close proximity, they become cross-linked, which interferes with protein synthesis and replication of the DNA in mitosis.

Cytotoxic Antibiotics

This second group of cell cycle phase non-specific drugs were originally developed as antibiotics, the majority from the *Streptomyces* fungus. So, some of these antibiotics, mainly the anthracyclines (a sub-group of these) and bleomycin, work on an enzyme called topoisomerase II. Topoisomerase II is an enzyme that works on the DNA double helix to help unravel the double helix in preparation for cell division (during the synthesis phase) and also helps in DNA repair (Figure 2.2). Anthracyclines block the action

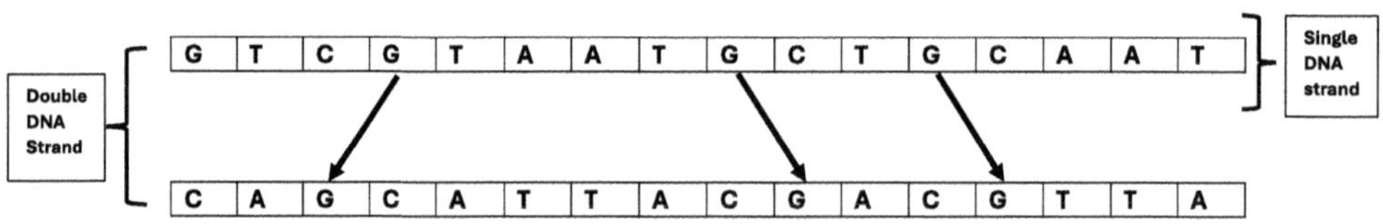

Figure 2.1 DNA strands with cross-linked guanine bases. Diagram of DNA strands with cross linked Guanine bases

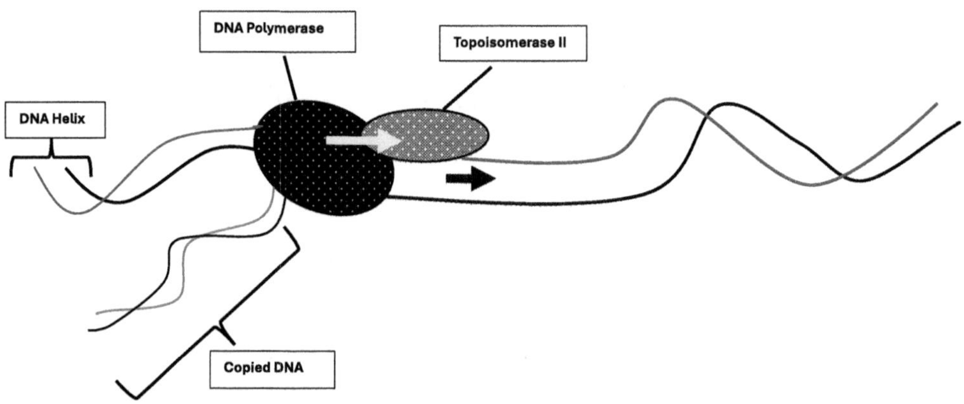

Figure 2.2 The normal action of the topoisomerase II enzyme. Diagram of the normal action of the topoisomerase II enzyme

of the topoisomerase II enzyme, rendering the cell unable to separate DNA strands and preventing DNA repair. This again causes DNA damage so that apoptosis is induced. Examples of anthracyclines are epirubicin, doxorubicin, daunorubicin and idarubicin (incidentally they are all quite brightly coloured drugs being mostly red/orange).

Other cytotoxic antibiotics include mitomycin, mitoxantrone (anthracycline derivative), bleomycin and dactinomycin. These drugs have slightly differing mechanisms of action. Dactinomycin binds to guanine – so similar in action to alkylating agents; mitomycin cross links the DNA bases in a similar way to alkylating agents; and bleomycin also produces free radicals which can fragment DNA (Chu and DeVita, 2020).

Topoisomerase Inhibitors

As described above, topoisomerase II inhibitors include doxorubicin, bleomycin and etoposide, but there are also topoisomerase I enzyme inhibitors such as irinotecan and topotecan. Topoisomerase I inhibitors create single DNA strand breaks preventing resealing and inhibiting replication, whereas topoisomerase II inhibitors create double DNA strand breaks, preventing chromosome separation during mitosis.

Cell Cycle Phase Specific Drugs

These drugs are only effective during specific parts or phases of the cell cycle (see Chapter 1). This means that only cells that are going through the designated phase will be affected by the drug, so it will only kill a proportion of cells in one go, unlike the cell cycle phase non-specific drugs. Therefore, these drugs tend to be given either over extended periods (for example in a pump over 46 hours or continuously in tablet form) or in divided doses (for example a short infusion every 12 hours) or are given frequently (for example weekly) to achieve a greater cell-killing effect. As with the cell cycle phase non-specific drugs, these can be further sub-categorised into the groups below.

Antimetabolites

These drugs prevent the formation of DNA bases that are required for DNA replication and repair. They do this by preventing the breakdown of amino acids into their constituent parts – DNA bases (See Figure 2.3). They are most active during the G1

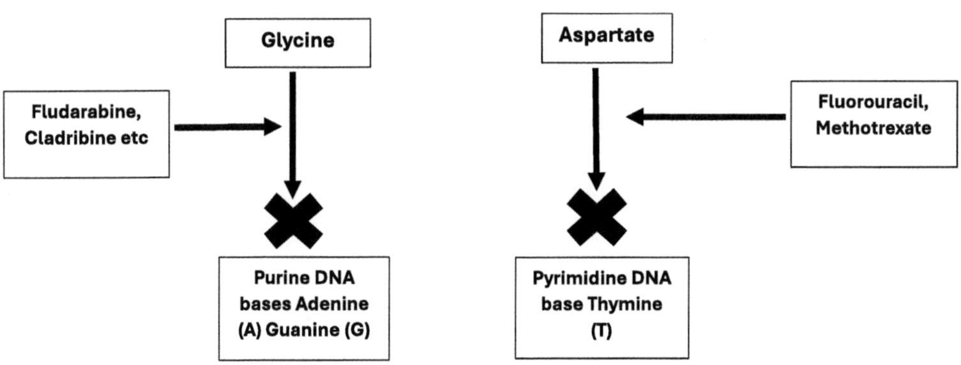

Figure 2.3 Action of antimetabolites

and S phases of the cell cycle because they prevent the formation of bases required for replication in the synthesis phase. Once the double helix splits open during S phase, allowing the corresponding bases to match up along the strand, as the bases required are not present in the cell, the strand cannot be replicated and therefore remains broken. This causes DNA damage which should be identified by the cell cycle checkpoint, and the cell should be put through apoptosis. If the cell has already completed the S phase of the cycle, the cell will not be damaged and therefore only a proportion of cells at any one time will be killed. Examples of antimetabolites include flourouracil (5Fu), methotraxate, cytarabine, fludarabine, gemcitibine, cladrabine and hydroxycarbamide.

Plant Alkaloids

This group of drugs mainly work during the mitotic phase of cell division as they affect the 'spindle', either by preventing it from forming by inhibiting tubulin production, or by locking the spindle into position, preventing the separation of chromosomes during mitosis. During cell division, a network of tubules forms across the cell, after the chromosomes are aligned into the centre of the cell during the metaphase of mitosis. This network is what allows the replicated chromosomes to separate and move to opposite poles of the cell before cytokinesis (physical splitting of the cell) takes place (Figure 2.4).

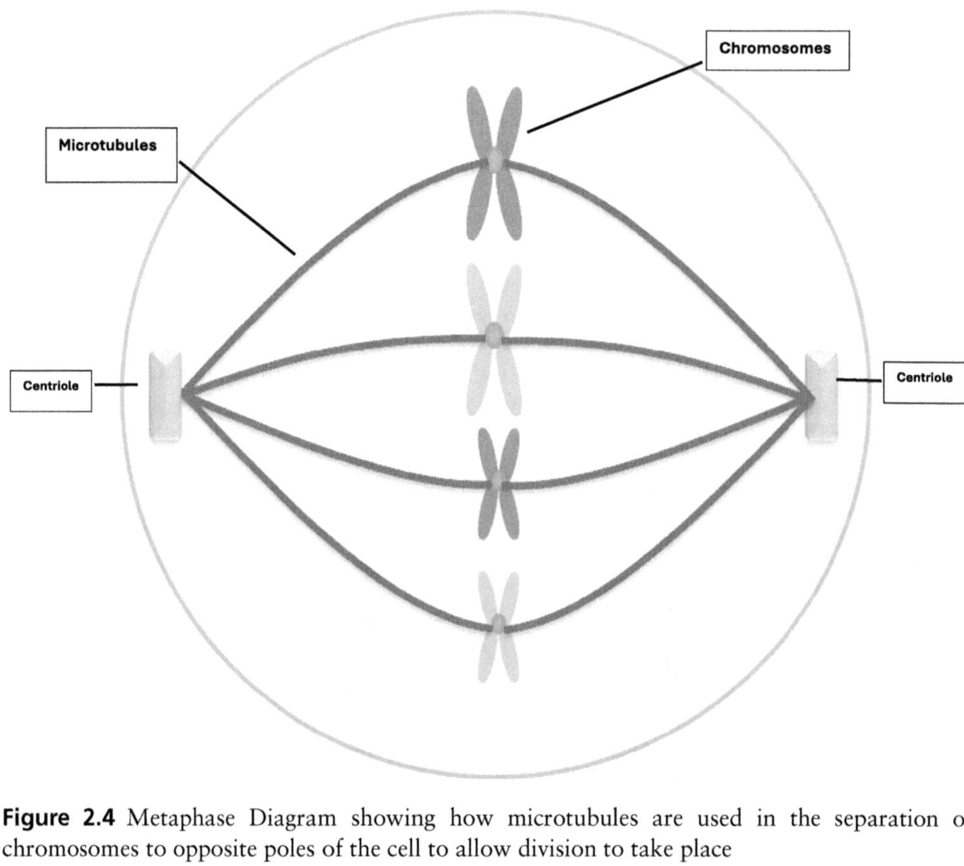

Figure 2.4 Metaphase Diagram showing how microtubules are used in the separation of chromosomes to opposite poles of the cell to allow division to take place

By preventing the formation of, or preventing the action of the spindle, the chromosomes cannot separate, and therefore the cell cannot divide. Examples of plant alkaloids include vincristine, vinblastine, vinorelbine, paclitaxel and docetaxel. All of these drugs originate from plants or are synthetic derivatives of them. Figure 2.4 shows how microtubules are used in the separation of chromosomes to opposite poles of the cell to allow division to take place.

Stop and Think ...

Can you explain how traditional chemotherapy drugs work and how this leads to the significant side effects that they cause?

Other SACT Types

There are numerous other SACT agents that do not specifically target cell replication. These drugs have been developed in more recent years and tend to either target intracellular signals, extracellular signals or block cell receptors that induce cell replication. These are discussed in much greater detail in Chapters 8 and 9; however, a brief outline is provided in Table 2.1

Combination SACT

The majority of SACT is given as a combination of different drugs as single agent treatments have never really evoked enough of a response to initiate a cure. Combining drugs maximises the cell-killing effect by using drugs that have different mechanisms of action, and that work on differing parts of the cell cycle. This also helps to prevent reaching the toxic effect of individual chemotherapy drugs – for example, platinum agents tend to be quite nephrotoxic (toxic to kidneys) and so the dose-limiting factor for these drugs tends to be related to renal function. However, if used in combination with an antimetabolite drug for example, the cell-killing effect is increased, but the nephrotoxicity is less likely to be reached as combining drugs has a similar effect to increasing the dose. Other groups of drugs tend to have other toxicities, for example anthracycline drugs can be cardiotoxic, plant alkaloids can cause quite severe peripheral neuropathy, and alkylating agents tend to be quite bone-marrow suppressive, while antimetabolites tend to effect mucous membranes causing sore mouth/eyes/skin (see Chapter 6).

The other reason for combining SACT agents is to reduce the risk of resistance to a particular chemotherapy drug. Cancer cells can build up resistance to chemotherapy over time; however, this is less likely when several drugs are used (Perry and Freter, 2012). Many years of clinical trials have enabled discovery of which drugs act best on which types of cancers, for example we know anthracyclines work well in breast cancers, and alkylating agents tend to work well in haematological cancers.

Aim of Treatment

SACT can be offered in a variety of ways – this can be with a curative intent, so for example a patient with breast cancer receiving adjuvant SACT (after surgery – to prevent disease recurrence) or neoadjuvant SACT (before surgery) where the likelihood

Table 2.1 An overview of other type of SACT, description and examples

SACT type	*Brief description*	*Examples*
Protein kinase inhibitors	Target intracellular pathways that allow cell replication to take place	Afatinib, axitinib, dasatinib, imatinib, osimertinib, niraparib, pazopanib, regorafenib, sorafenib, sunitinib
Proteosome inhibitors	Cause a build-up of these proteins which can subsequently become toxic to the cell and induce apoptosis	Bortezomib, carfilzomib, ixazomib
Targeted biotherapies	Engineered antibodies to target the receptor -blocking a growth factor from landing on the receptor, thus preventing replication of the cancer cell	Trastuzumab, pertuzumab, rituximab, obinituzumab
Antibody-Drug Conjugates (ADCs)	Monoclonal Antibodies attached to cytotoxic chemotherapy agents	Trastuzumab emtansine, trastuzumab deruxtecan, enfortumab vedotin
Immunotherapy	Monoclonal antibodies that are engineered to harness the immune systems' effects on cancer and enhance destruction of cancer cells by the patient's own immune system	Nivolumab, pembrolizumab, ipilimumab
Hormone antagonists	Hormone treatments used in theprevention and treatment of hormone mediated cancers such as breast cancer and prostate cancer	Anastrozole, letrozole, exemestane bicalutamide, cyproterone, abiraterone, enzalutamide, daralutamide and apalutamide
CDK4/6 inhibitors	Target and inhibit Cyclin-Dependent Kinases (CDK) 4 and 6- critical regulators of the cell cycle particularly between G1 and S phases of the cycle	Palbociclib, abemaciclib, ribociclib
PARP inhibitors	PARP (Poly ADP Ribose Polymerase) is an enzyme that is engaged in DNA repair, therefore inhibition of this enzyme can lead to apoptosis	Olaparib, niraparib, rucaparib

is that the patient will be cancer-free after their whole treatment pathway. SACT can be given before surgery (neoadjuvant) with the aim of shrinking down the cancer size, improving success of the subsequent surgery. When SACT is given in the adjuvant setting (after a different treatment such as surgery or radiotherapy) the aim is to reduce the risk of recurrence by eliminating any remaining malignant cells that may have been left behind, as there is no way of knowing if one or two malignant cells have made their way into the circulation/lymphatic system to potentially create metastasis further down the line. Many haematological cancers are also treated with a curative intent as SACT alone can have a significant impact on these diseases as they tend to respond better to treatment due to the rate of cell division.

SACT can also be given alongside radiotherapy (often referred to as chemo-rad treatment), for example in patients with head and neck cancers, whereby a combination of the two types of treatment together can produce very good results and sometimes cure.

Alternatively (and for many patients that are treated with SACT) treatment can be given with a palliative intent. This means that we are unlikely to be able to cure the patient; they will not be cancer-free, but good results can be obtained by shrinking cancers thus reducing symptoms and preventing further disease progression, consequently potentially prolonging life. Some patients now can receive palliative treatment for significant time periods – some of them for many years, hence there is a shift towards cancer as more of a long-term condition and emphasis around living with and beyond cancer. Consistent developments in treatment mean that patients are living for much longer, even with non-curative cancers.

It is important to understand the aim of treatment at the outset, as chemotherapy can have a massive impact and patients all respond very differently. For example, if the aim is curative, there is less room for alterations in the regime as the longer-term outcomes can become affected – especially with neoadjuvant and adjuvant treatments – the aim is always to adhere to the planned dosing and schedule unless the patient has severe toxicity, in which case the regime may have to be amended or reconsidered. However, if the patient is receiving SACT with palliative intent, it is more of a balancing act to ensure that side effects do not impact heavily on the patient's quality of life, but maintains an active response on disease, reducing symptoms and improving their progression-free survival.

Example Regimen

It may be useful to look at a commonly used SACT regime to help understand how the drugs are put together, and how this can enhance the impact on disease and improve outcomes. The CHOP chemotherapy regime has been used for many years in the treatment of Non-Hodgkins Lymphoma (NHL) disease. In general, the acronym refers to the first letter of each drug in the regime so in this case, C-Cyclophosphamide, H- Doxorubicin (formerly known as Hydroxydaunorubicin), O-Vincristine (formerly known as Oncovin®) and P-Prednisolone.

Cyclophosphamide is an alkylating agent, so cell cycle non-phase specific, having a big overall cell-killing effect. It tends to be fairly bone-marrow suppressive, with bladder toxicity possible in high doses. Doxorubicin (the 'H' in CHOP) is an anthracycline, cytotoxic antibiotic. Again, cell cycle phase non-specific, so it also has a large overall cell-killing effect while also bone-marrow suppressive; one of its main toxicities is cardiotoxicity, and it also needs to be dose-adjusted in patients with reduced liver function.

Vincristine is a plant alkaloid, so is cell cycle phase specific (affecting mitosis by preventing spindle formation), so will only affect cells that are in the mitotic phase; however, as the target in this case is overproduction of B-cells (a type of white blood cell), vincristine is likely to have significant impact due to the rapid proliferation of these cells and thus significant numbers in the mitotic phase. The toxicity that is most associated with vincristine is peripheral neuropathy (deadening of nerve endings in hands/feet) (Chu and DeVita, 2020).

Prednisolone in this regime is used to stimulate resting cells in G0 phase to the active phase of the cell cycle (G1) and thus makes them more susceptible to the action of the cytotoxic drugs in the regime.

So overall, the regime combines different drugs with different mechanisms of action, all of which have differing toxicities, therefore making it less likely that a significant toxicity would be reached as the combination of drugs together has a synergistic effect allowing the dosing of drugs to be given at an optimal level that reduces the risk of reaching a specific toxicity.

Spotlight on Cancer Treatment

Since around 2009, there has been enhanced scrutiny on the appropriateness of SACT – how it is given, who it is given to, and the management of toxicity. This is due to a report that was produced in that year which was a NCEPOD (National Confidential Enquiry into Patient Outcomes and Deaths) and subsequent report (National Chemotherapy Advisory Group (NCAG), 2009) which looked at over 600 patient records that were receiving SACT. The report found that there were significant improvements that needed to be made – particularly around the fitness level of patients receiving treatment, their awareness of the possible outcomes/risks and the appropriate management of specific toxicities. The Acute Oncology Service was born because of this report, but there were additional guidelines relating to patient consent, fitness to treat, and an investigation into any patient's death within 30 days of receiving SACT. These guidelines are currently upheld and so all trusts where SACT is delivered should have an Acute Oncology service and should also have a monthly Mortality and Morbidity meeting where deaths within 30 days of SACT are discussed, along with any significant morbidities as a result of patients receiving SACT. Patients should also have a regular assessment of their fitness to receive treatment, usually in the form of a World Health Organisation (WHO) Performance status score, combined with blood results falling within specific parameters for the particular regime and a full assessment of any SACT-related toxicities.

Summary

This chapter has detailed the mechanisms of action of a variety of SACT, how they are put together into regimes, and how they impact on different types of cancers. Having an understanding of this can aid healthcare practitioners when managing patients receiving SACT so that they can explain how the drugs may impact them, why they are given in the way that they are, and how the potential side effects are caused. This enables healthcare professionals in providing appropriate and accurate information that will aid in obtaining informed consent prior to commencing SACT.

Stop and Think ...

Would you be able to explain a complete SACT regime to a patient including how it works and its side effects?

References

Chu, E. and DeVita, V.T. (2020) *Physicians' cancer chemotherapy drug manual 2020*. Burlington, MA: Jones and Bartlett learning.

McFadden, R. (2019) *Introducing pharmacology for nursing and healthcare*. 3rd Edition. Oxon: Routledge.

National Chemotherapy Advisory Group (NCAG, 2009) *Chemotherapy services in England: Ensuring quality and safety*. A report from the National Chemotherapy Advisory Group AUGUST 2009, available at: [ARCHIVED CONTENT]

Perry, M.C. and Freter, C.E. (2012) *Perry's the chemotherapy source book*. 5th Edition. Philidelphia: Lippincott Williams and Wilkins.

CHAPTER 3

Extravasation

Samantha Toland

Introduction

Extravasation is a complication that can occur when administering IV Systemic Anti-Cancer Treatment (SACT). It is classed as an emergency due to the potential for serious consequences and injuries, so prevention and immediate management are essential. Any healthcare professional administering SACT should know how to manage this complication effectively to avoid a serious injury from occurring and needs to adhere to the policies and protocols in place within their area of work due to the risk of litigation should a serious injury occur.

What is Extravasation?

Definitions

Extravasation is the inadvertent administration of vesicant drugs outside of the venous path and into the surrounding tissues which can lead to tissue damage and necrosis. The main difference between extravasation and infiltration is that an extravasation generally refers to the use of vesicant drugs, whereas infiltration usually refers to non-vesicant drugs. So what do we mean by vesicant drugs? A vesicant drug is any solution or medication that can cause blistering, sloughing of tissues and tissue necrosis when administered outside of the venous path (Perez-Fidalgo et al., 2012). Within oncology and haemato-oncology we generally refer to this when administering a cytotoxic (a cell-killing type of SACT) vesicant drug. There are a range of vesicant cytotoxic drugs used within these areas including vincristine, doxorubin, paclitaxel and epirubicin to name just a few.

Drugs can be categorised according to their vesicant/irritant properties as shown in Table 3.1 below:

DOI: 10.4324/9781003516477-3

Table 3.1 Table of Vesicant Chemotherapy Drugs

Vesicants	*Irritants*	*Non-Vesicants*
DNA-Binding:	Bendamustine	Arsenic trioxide
Amsacrine	Carboplatin	Asparaginase
Carmustine	Cisplatin	Bleomycin
Dacarbazine	Etoposide	Bortezomib
Dactinomycin	Fluorouracil	Cladrabine
Daunorubicin	Ifosfamide	Cyclophosphamide
Doxorubicin	Irinotecan	Cytarabine
Epirubicin	Liposomal daunorubicin	Eribulin
Idarubicin	Liposomal doxorubicin	Fludarabine
Mechlorethamine	Melphalan	Gemcitabine
(Nitrogen Mustard/Mustine)	Methotrexate	Monoclonal antibodies
Mitomycin	Mitoxantrone	Paclitaxel albumin
Streptozocin	Oxaliplatin	Pemetrexed
Treosulphan	Temsirolimus	Pentostatin
	Teniposide	Raltitrexed
Non-DNA-Binding:	Topotecan	Thiotepa
Cabazitaxel	Trastuzumab emtansine	
Docetaxel	(Kadcyla)	
Paclitaxel	Aflibercept	
Trabectedin		
Vinblastine		
Vincristine		
Vindesine		
Vinflunine		
Vinorelbine		

What Can Happen as a Result of Extravasation?

Extravasation injuries can range from an almost insignificant reaction such as an area of redness and/or swelling, to severe injury with tissue necrosis which may eventually require surgical intervention such as skin grafting. The difficulty in identifying and grading an extravasation injury is the fact that it is progressive and so the extent of damage may not materialise for weeks, sometimes even months. These injuries, depending on how deeply they penetrate the tissue, could then involve internal structures such as tendons, nerves and potentially even joints can become affected.

Figure 3.1 shows a picture of an extravasation injury resulting from the extravasation of a vesicant cytotoxic drug. You can see an area of sloughing in the middle where the tissue is yellow in colour, and the surrounding darker tissue is where the area is starting to necrose. This clearly demonstrates the impact of having an extravasation injury. This will significantly impact quality of life and potential ability to carry out normal activities of daily living.

Fortunately, in more recent years severe extravasation injuries are much less common. This is mostly due to heightened awareness, better prevention including

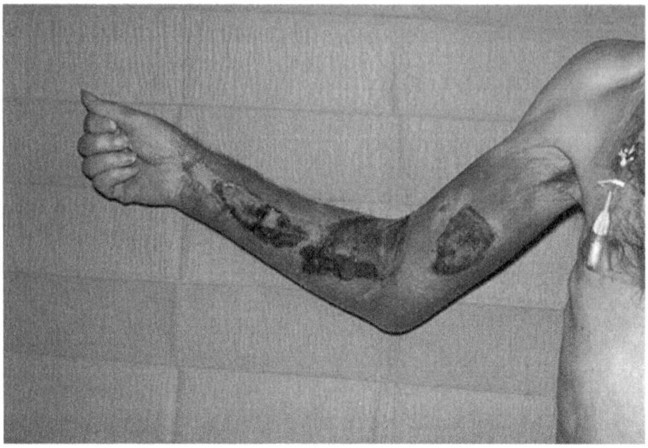

Figure 3.1 Hand extravasation injury in a patient

improved cannulation technique/devices, earlier recognition and prompt management of extravasation at the time of administration resulting in smaller and less severe injuries (Olver, 2018).

Risk Factors

There are a number of risk factors which can contribute to the potential for an extravasation to occur. These include choice of cannulation site, equipment factors, patient factors (such as age and comorbidities), healthcare professional factors, environmental factors and concurrent medications/order of administration of drugs; these will now be explored in more detail.

Cannulation/IV Site

Ideally the first choice for cannulation should always be between wrist and elbow (but not at the site of any joints) (Perez-Fidalgo, 2012). This is for a couple of reasons; one being that this part of the arm acts a natural splint – there is very little movement possible even if the hands are in motion, reducing the risk of a cannula becoming dislodged. Secondly, if an extravasation injury were to occur in this part of the arm, the longer-term damage would likely have a lesser impact on quality of life as it is less likely to affect fine motor movement in the hand. There is generally more subcutaneous fat and tissue present, preventing the injury from affecting deeper nerve/tendon tissues. Cannulation can be performed in the back of the hand, but this should not be the first choice of IV site for reasons specified above, i.e. if the healthcare practitioner cannot identify an appropriate vein for cannulation in the arm but can see a suitable vein in the back of the hand, this may be the most appropriate site in this instance, but this would need to be justified within the documentation (as described later in this chapter).

Ideally when administering vesicant drugs a fresh IV site should be used, i.e. a new cannula placed immediately before administration of the drugs because the integrity of the vein is at its best. It is also ideal that the healthcare practitioner administering the drug is the same person who cannulates the patient as they can be certain of the cannula placement and feel confident that this was performed appropriately for administration of vesicant medications.

Equipment

When cannulating for SACT and particularly when there are vesicant drugs in a regime, it is important to use the smallest device feasible, so this would be either a 23- or 24-gauge cannula. The rationale for this is to obtain an adequate blood flow around the device which helps to prevent both chemical and mechanical phlebitis which can result when either the drug or device has sustained contact with the vein walls.

Central venous access devices (CVADs) are often used for administration of SACT (see Chapter 10), as they have several advantages over peripheral cannulation – one of these being additional safety in administration of vesicant SACT. This is because CVADs are long-term catheters that are much less likely to become damaged/dislodged so are most appropriate for administration of vesicant SACT. However, there remains a risk of extravasation so it is paramount that CVADs are checked prior to administration to ensure patency of the line. This may involve checking for back flow of blood through the device by withdrawing from the CVAD using a 10 ml syringe, and for a lack of resistance when flushing with solutions. If back flow is absent or flushing becomes sluggish, an X-ray may be required to check that the tip of the device remains in the appropriate placement before proceeding with administration of vesicant SACT.

Patient Factors

There are several patient factors that need to be taken into consideration – these include:

- Comorbidities
  Other conditions such as hypertension, diabetes, peripheral vascular disease, cardiovascular disease and vascular impairment (e.g. Raynaud's disease) can all have an impact on the risk of extravasation. Any condition that may affect the integrity or quality of the veins in the extremities will increase the risk of extravasation.
- Age
  There are no limitations to age when it comes to people receiving SACT, unless their performance status/frailty level indicates that treatment would be inappropriate. However, the older a person is, the more fragile their veins become so they are generally more at risk of an extravasation. Older people are also more likely to have comorbidities and be receiving multiple medications as a result, so are at a higher risk of extravasation for several reasons.
- Disease-related factors
  Some patients with certain types of cancer may have a complication known as lymphedema – this is where either from surgical intervention or from the disease itself (e.g. lymphoma), the lymphatic drainage becomes affected, and this can increase the risk of extravasation. This is because vesicant drugs can remain within the venous path for much longer than normal increasing the risk of chemical phlebitis and therefore extravasation. Many patients with breast cancer have issues with lymphedema and this often means it is favourable to use the unaffected arm for treatment. However, multiple cannulations and administration of vesicants into one arm can also increase the risk of extravasation – so it is often advisable to use CVADs in these circumstances.

- Concurrent medications
  Concurrent medications can potentially impact the risk of extravasation, for example, patients receiving antihypertensive drugs in the form of calcium channel blockers – these medications cause vasodilation to reduce central venous pressure and subsequently reduce blood pressure thus potentially increasing the amount of drug that extravasates into an area. Other drugs such as antihistamines and steroids can also affect the integrity of the venous path by causing vasoconstriction, vasodilation or by reducing any inflammatory reaction in an area of extravasation and therefore potentially masking the symptoms of this.
- Communication barriers
  Patients need to be made fully aware of the risks, signs and symptoms of extravasation in order that they can communicate when an extravasation may be taking place. Therefore, patients need to be able to report any signs such as pain, stinging or changes at the infusion site. If there are any barriers to communicating this information, this must be documented and the patient closely monitored throughout the administration.
- Venous access issues
  It is always advisable for patients to have a CVAD if they are due to commence SACT which contains vesicant drugs – particularly patients who have poor venous access before they have commenced treatment. Multiple attempts at venepuncture and cannulation significantly increase the risk of extravasation. It is imperative that any additional attempts at cannulation for treatment are undertaken above previous puncture sites as there is a risk that the drug may leak out of the vein (WMCA Guidelines, 2024).

Order of Drug Administration

As detailed above, there are medications that can affect the integrity of the venous path – this also applies when administering any SACT regime. Most SACT protocols involve administration of antiemetics and/or steroids intravenously prior to administration of SACT, however if vesicant drugs are part of the regime these should always be given first. This is because the vein is at optimal integrity when freshly cannulated so this is the best point in time to use that vein for vesicant administration. Additionally, other drugs that are administered can cause site reactions, for example, ondansetron can induce a flare reaction, causing redness to appear at the site of administration which can mistakenly be diagnosed as extravasation; steroids can potentially mask signs of extravasation because this could prevent inflammation at the administration site. (N.B. if these pre-medications are to be administered orally, they can be given in advance of the SACT.) If pre-medications are required specifically to be administered before the SACT (such as antihistamines/steroids with the aim of preventing a reaction) then these should be given prior to any SACT, however the practitioner should bear in mind that this may potentially increase the risk of an extravasation.

Healthcare Professional Competency and Skill

It is imperative that healthcare practitioners who administer SACT have the appropriate level of background knowledge and understanding, but also the level of clinical skill and competence in terms of being able to cannulate effectively and administer vesicant drugs. Administration of vesicant drugs can be a difficult task because there are so many different factors to consider, and multiple aspects to focus on – constant observation of the cannula site, communication to provide reassurance to the patient, and concentration to ensure the drugs are being given correctly and in accordance with the SACT protocol. Anyone administering vesicant medications should also be fully aware of what action to take should an extravasation occur. This is why it is important for healthcare practitioners to have been deemed competent following a training and competency programme in practice before administering SACT independently.

Patient Education

Patient education is paramount to ensure safe administration of vesicant SACT and should be an ongoing process from consent through to administration and after completion of SACT. Patients should be made aware of the risks associated with extravasation during consent, and this should again be reiterated during the pre-SACT consultation process. They should also be informed of what to look out for during administration of the drugs, i.e. any redness, stinging, swelling or changes in sensation, and this should again be reiterated when patients attend for treatment.

Guidelines

All healthcare professionals administering SACT need to ensure that they adhere strictly to policies and protocols in order that their employer can provide vicarious liability for any legal action taken as a result of an extravasation injury. There should be an extravasation policy in place in any area where SACT is administered which all healthcare practitioners should be familiar with before administering vesicant drugs.

Administration of Vesicant SACT

There are several techniques that can be applied to administration of vesicant drugs which can help to reduce the risk and severity of an extravasation. Vesicant drugs should always be given concurrently with a fast-flowing infusion of an appropriate diluting solution (usually saline). This is so that the vesicant drug becomes diluted, reducing the concentration of the drug as it enters the vein, reducing the risk of extravasation or severe injury/harm should an extravasation occur. This can be done by administering the vesicant drug through the side arm of an administration set while a free-flowing solution is in progress, or by use of specialist administration pumps whereby the vesicant is attached to the pump to be given alongside a concurrent line of fast-flowing solution.

The cannula site should be checked regularly and the device checked for patency. This can be done by drawing back on the syringe while occluding the administration line to obtain a back flow of blood, confirming the cannula remains within the venous path if being administered by hand, or by pausing the administration through a pump and lowering the bag of solution below waist height enabling a back flow of blood into the line via gravity. For either method, this check should be carried out prior to administration of a vesicant and then regularly throughout administration. The cannula site must remain clear so that it can be freely observed – therefore transparent cannula dressings must be applied and any securing tape must not impede the ability to see the site clearly. The use of bandages or coverings to secure cannula sites must be avoided.

If there is any doubt about the patency of the cannula it should be immediately removed and another one placed proximally to the previous site.

The cannula site should be constantly observed for any signs of redness/swelling and the drips within the administration set chamber monitored to ensure there is an easy flow of solution, with no resistance/slowing down of the drip rate. Specialist administration pumps can be set to detect minimal changes in pressure, and it is recommended that sensors be set to detect very low-pressure changes when administering vesicant drugs peripherally.

Use of CVADs can reduce the risk of extravasation as they are more robust in general than using a peripheral cannula – however it should be noted that the risk of extravasation remains with CVADs, so it is imperative that their patency is checked effectively before use with vesicant drugs and that there is no pain/discomfort when administering via a CVAD.

Signs and Symptoms of Extravasation

So, what might we see when an extravasation happens? There may be some indication of an extravasation taking place during administration in the form of sudden resistance/lack of flow of infusion solution, or lack of blood return during checks. There might be signs and symptoms of pain, burning or stinging at the cannula site. However, some vesicant drugs may cause stinging and tingling at the site anyway due to their caustic properties, so it is important to be able to differentiate between extravasation and other venous effects. There may be some redness, swelling and/or tenderness at the site, and possibly venous discolouration, but some vesicant drugs cause venous discoloration because they are often brightly coloured, again emphasising the importance of being able to differentiate between extravasation and other events.

It is important to note that occasionally there are very few/no symptoms evident during an extravasation and that there is the possibility of a partial cannula displacement whereby the tip of the cannula is part placed in the vein, part within the tissue (Roe, 2016). In this scenario, the drugs appear to be flowing into the venous path as blood return tends to remain evident, however some of the drug is allowed to escape into the surrounding tissue resulting in an extravasation. This is much more difficult to identify and therefore less likely to be managed immediately potentially resulting in a more severe injury

Other Vessel Reactions

Flare Reaction

A flare reaction can occur when a drug creates a reaction causing local histamine release resulting in red blotches/hives around the administration site, sometimes tracking up the arm. This can happen with a variety of drugs, one of these drugs being ondansetron (anti-emetic drug). Flare reactions usually appear quite rapidly from the onset of giving the drug itself and tend to resolve quickly. The only way to diagnose a flare reaction is to stop administration of the drug and to let the site settle down for around 30–45 minutes.

If at that time the redness starts to dissipate and the site is almost back to normal, the likelihood is a flare reaction. Swelling is rarely present, and blood return usually remains intact.

Vessel Irritation

Many SACT drugs can cause vessel irritation, simply by virtue of their pH values – many of them being either acidic or alkaline. Patients often feel aching and tightness along the vein and that can sometimes be accompanied by some redness/erythema or discolouration along the vessel. This tends to happen near the beginning of administration of the drug, and swelling is unlikely. Blood return usually remains intact, but it may be that if the vessel irritation has caused the vein to spasm, then blood return may temporarily be absent.

Vessel Spasm

Some SACT drugs can cause the vessel to go into spasm – particularly if they are very cold. As vein walls are mostly made of muscle tissue, they can easily go into spasm following contact with drugs or cold temperatures. This causes the pressure within the vessel to increase resulting in a reduction in the flow of infusion fluid, and blood return may cease. This can also cause issues when administering via infusion pumps as the pressure increases in the vessel causing the pump to alarm. Applying heat can sometimes help, however care should be taken to ensure heat is applied away from the cannula site so if redness appears this is not mistaken for extravasation or flare reaction. Vessel spasm tends to appear immediately on administration of the drug and other symptoms such as discoloration or swelling in the site are unlikely.

Differentiation of Venous Reactions

The only event that is likely to have most of the presenting symptoms described above is an extravasation. So, pain, burning and stinging is common at the cannula/CVAD entry site; there tends to be redness and/or swelling around the site; blood return tends to either be sluggish or disappears. However definitive diagnosis can be difficult, and it is useful to ask a colleague to come and review the site to be able to confirm what the most likely cause of the symptoms is. If there is any concern or suspicion that an extravasation has occurred, it must be acted upon immediately and treated as an emergency.

Management of Extravasation

Extravasation is an oncological and haemato-oncology emergency, so it is imperative to act quickly. If an extravasation injury is suspected chemotherapy administration should be stopped immediately, and the extravasation kit straight should be sought right away (these kits should be available in all areas where SACT is administered (see example of kit below). Assistance will be required to manage the event so calling for colleagues to help is essential, as it tends to be distressing for the staff administering the drugs and therefore support in the management of the extravasation is needed.

The first step in the management of the extravasation is to attach an empty syringe and aspirate from the cannula or CVAD. This is performed to try and undo the harm that has been potentially made by the extravasation – by withdrawing as much of the offending drug as possible. The area should then be marked with an indelible pen so that the site can be monitored for any changes. A digital image can also be taken (provided the patient has given consent to do so (see Chapter 4)), again to allow for adequate monitoring of any changes to the site. A decision then needs to be made regarding the appropriate treatment, which will depend upon the type of drug that has been extravasated.

There are two main classifications of vesicant drugs: those which are DNA binding, and those that are non-DNA binding (see Table 3.1). It is important to understand this in order to carry out the appropriate management as they are managed very differently.

DNA-Binding Drugs

These drugs bind to the DNA within the cells of the tissues during extravasation (see Chapter 2). This means that they destroy the cells within the dermis layer surrounding the site, but as these drugs tend to have a longer half-life within the tissues, they are then released to the subsequent layer and so on, creating progressive tissue necrosis. For this reason, the principle for management of an extravasation of these drugs is to localise and neutralise. This can be done by firstly administering a cold pack to the area to cause vasoconstriction, thus restricting any further spread of the drug within the tissues. Secondly, an antidote may be administered depending on the specific drug involved or alternatively plastic surgery techniques such as saline flush out may be performed if this is available within the local area (see Figure 3.2). Antidotes available for DNA-binding drugs include DMSO (dimethyl sulphoxide) and dexrazoxane (Savene). DMSO is a topical treatment that needs to be delivered within two hours of the extravasation, and which requires further applications every two hours for the first 24 hours, then every six hours for up to seven days after. DMSO is thought to have properties of scavenging free radicals in the tissue, reducing the tissue damage due to extravasation. In general, this tends to be used for smaller size extravasation injuries (<3 mls in size) (Perez-Fidalgo 2012).

Dexrazoxane (Savene) is an intravenous cytotoxic drug and is the only licenced antidote for extravasation of anthracycline drugs (daunorubicin, doxorubicin, epirubicin, idarubicin). It needs to be used within six hours of the extravasation and is given as a one-hour infusion daily for three days. It blocks the action of the anthracycline drug within the tissues, preventing injury as a result of extravasation. It is the only pharmacological method of management that shows efficacy in biopsy-confirmed anthracycline extravasation that has been confirmed in clinical trials. Cold packs must be removed at least 15 minutes before use of dexrazoxane to ensure the drug is not prevented from entering the extravasation area due to local vasoconstriction. Additional venous access must be sought for administration, and as it is a cytotoxic drug, it carries similar side effects/toxicities to other SACT so these need to be monitored for.

N.B. DMSO and dexrazoxane should not be used concurrently.

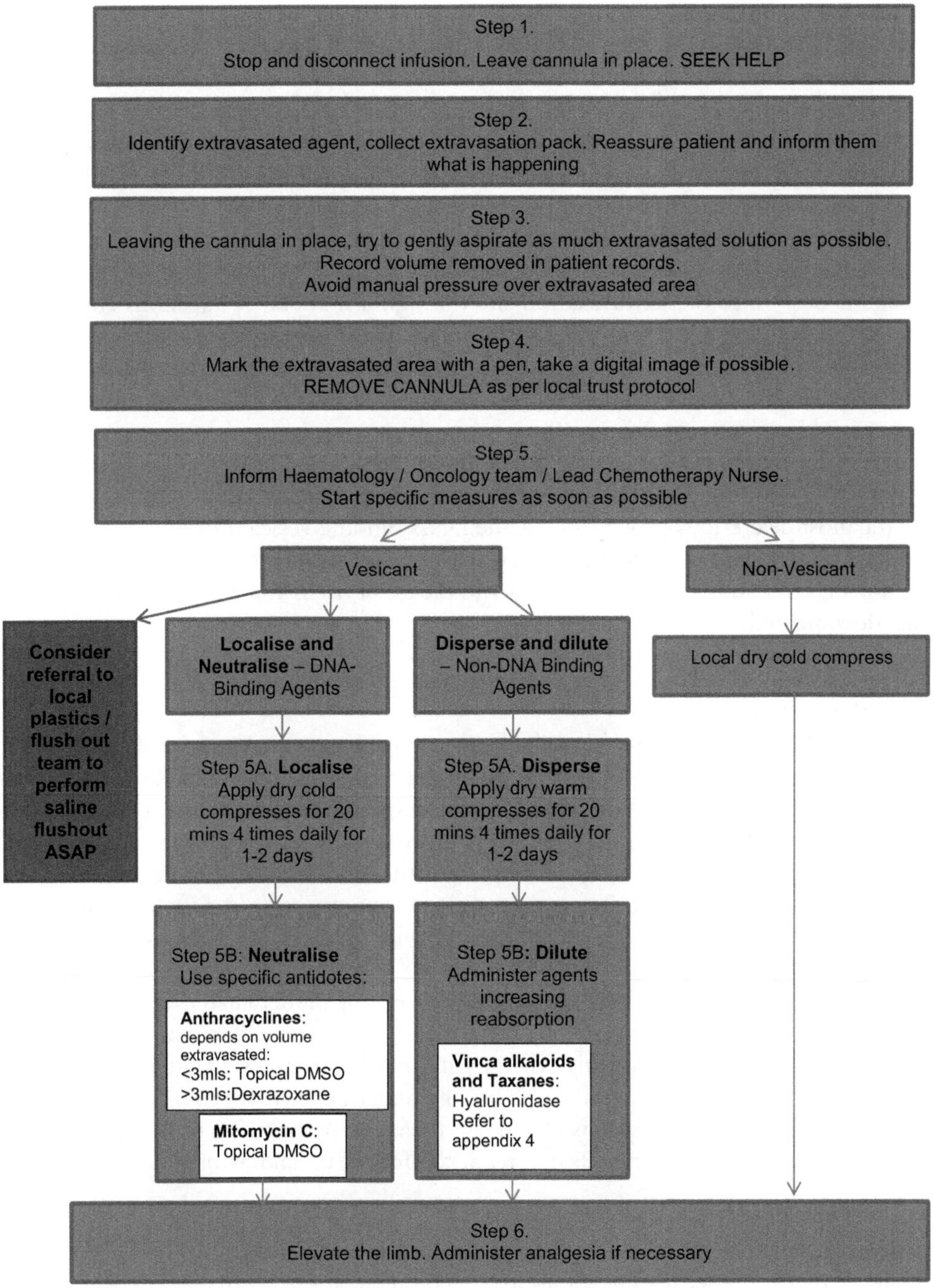

Figure 3.2 Management of extravasation via peripheral cannula flow chart

Non-DNA-Binding Drugs

Non-DNA-binding drugs don't generally cause as much damage to the tissues, as they tend to be metabolised within the tissue and therefore do not tend to cause necrosis as their DNA-binding counterparts do. They can cause injury, but this tends to be more in the form of blistering, much like a burn. This means the principle of management is different for this group of drugs and it is appropriate to spread and dilute the extravasated drug. This involves use of a warm pack to aid vasodilation of the extravasated area – this helps to encourage the extravasated drug back into the venous path, and dilution/dispersal of the drug is obtained by use of hyaluronidase. Hyaluronidase is administered subcutaneously into the extravasation site through a number of injections covering at least the four compass points around the area. This breaks down collagen fibres in the tissues, allowing the extravasated drug to disperse more freely in the tissue, and as the vessels are dilated through use of the warm compress, the extravasated drug is encouraged back into circulation.

N.B. if the extravasation has the possibility of being from both a DNA-binding and/or non-DNA-binding drug, treatment should be given in accordance with the drug that has the most deleterious properties, i.e. the DNA-binding vesicant drug.

Once appropriate treatment has been delivered, the patient will require additional monitoring over subsequent days/weeks and the event needs to be very clearly and carefully documented.

Surgical Intervention

There are also surgical methods available to manage extravasation injuries, such as the saline flush-out technique. This involves making several incisions within the extravasated area, inserting a cannula into the subcutaneous tissue and flushing the area through with saline. This technique is used to completely flush out the SACT from the tissue to prevent an extravasation injury from developing further and is performed in several centres within the United Kingdom. Referral to a plastic surgery team is usually required for this – however many centres are unable to provide this service if they do not have a plastic surgery team on site.

Treatment of unresolved tissue necrosis or pain lasting more than ten days may involve surgical debridement; this is generally for patients who have suffered a severe extravasation injury in whom conservative therapy has not been appropriately initiated. Once this has been performed, skin grafting is usually undertaken. This again requires referral to a plastic surgery team – this is effectively managed by referring in the initial stages of an extravasation so that the plastics team can follow up and manage as appropriate.

Evidence Base

While there are numerous guidelines and recommendations available regarding management of extravasation, there is very little evidence to support them. This is due to the diverse nature of extravasation incidents making randomised controlled trials extremely difficult, and often multiple management strategies are applied, making it impossible to determine how successful individual treatments are. There are also no direct comparator studies looking at surgical versus pharmacological management strategies, so it can depend upon individual circumstances and clinical decision-making as to applying the most appropriate strategy for management (Thomas et al., 2025).

Documentation

Accurate and timely documentation of an extravasation is paramount due to the likelihood of litigation following a severe injury. It is also important to document the steps taken to prevent an extravasation, so whoever has administered the vesicant SACT can demonstrate that they have performed in line with current best practice and protocol guidelines. Documentation should include:

- Patient name and number
- Clinical area
- Date and time of extravasation
- Name of drug which has extravasated
- Signs and symptoms
  - Colour of surrounding skin
  - Size of extravasation
- Description of the IV access
  - Venepuncture site
  - Size and position of cannula
  - Number of attempts at obtaining venous access and positions
  - Drugs administered and the sequence
  - Drug administration technique (bolus or infusion)
  - Blood return
- Extravasation area
  - Approximate amount of the drug extravasated
  - Photograph of extravasated area
  - Size (diameter, length and width) of extravasation area
  - Appearance of extravasation area
- Step-by-step management with date and time of each step performed and medical notification
  - Aspiration possible (including amount) or not, location (venous and/or subcutaneous) and amount
  - Cold/heat
  - Antidote
  - Referral details (if any)
- Patient's complaints, comments, statements
- Indication that patient's information sheet given to patient
- Follow-up instructions given (to patient, nurse, physician, etc.)
- Names of all professionals involved in the patient management
- Signature of nurse

All follow-up care should be documented in the notes, and all visual assessments should be recorded (WMCA Guideline, 2024).

Patient Information

Patients should be provided with an information leaflet detailing what will happen after an extravasation has taken place – what to look out for, and how they will be followed up in the subsequent days/weeks.

Follow Up

Follow-up must be provided after an extravasation has occurred; this would usually involve a review of the site daily for the first few days, then every 3–7 days up to the next cycle of treatment. Plastic surgery team may also be involved as part of the follow up so they can monitor for any signs of tissue breakdown/necrosis and can act upon this quickly.

Staff Support

It can be quite distressing for the staff member involved in an extravasation as no healthcare professional sets out to cause harm to a patient, and it can be anxiety-provoking to be in that situation. It is imperative that they are provided with support, both in the management of the extravasation, but also after the event and it is good practice to debrief and reflect on the incident.

Example Extravasation Kit

- Copy of extravasation guideline (also available on the intranet)
- 10 ml syringes
- Green needles, orange needles
- Water for injection
- Alcohol wipes
- Sterile gauze and cotton wool
- Cold and hot packs (available within chemotherapy units)
- Hyaluronidase 1500 units x 2
- DMSO
- Hydrocortisone 1% cream labelled with instructions for use to reduce local trauma and irritation
- Non-occlusive dressing
- Savene kit (available in aseptic suite)

Summary

This chapter has outlined the prevention strategies, recognition, and management of extravasations in relation to administration of SACT. It highlights the importance of patient education and staff competency in administration of vesicant SACT so that prompt recognition and management can take place as this is recognised as an emergency situation, so immediate response is essential. Healthcare professionals administering vesicant SACT should know the specific management strategies required for the drugs they are giving and should always work to local policies/protocols to ensure that they are providing the most appropriate care for patients undergoing this type of treatment.

References

Olver, I. (ed) (2018) 'Extravasation', in *The MASCC Textbook of Cancer Supportive Care and Survivorship*. 2nd Edition. Springer International Publishing AG. Switzerland, pp. 587–596.

Perez-Fidalgo, J.A., Garcia Fabregat, L., Cervantes, A., Marguiles, A., Vidall, C., Roila, F. and on behalf of the ESMO Guidelines working group (2012) Management of chemotherapy extravasation: ESMO-EONS clinical practice guidelines. *European Journal of Oncology Nursing*, 16, 528–534.

Roe, H. (2016) *Managing chemotherapy extravasations in practice*. Hospital Pharmacy Europe, available at: https://hospitalpharmacyeurope.com/clinical-zones/oncology/managing-chemotherapy-extravasations-in-practice/

Thomas, T., Clark, C., Backler, C., Bohlke, K., Centofanti, D., Jotwani, A.C., Cope, D.G., Dalton, K.A., Gochett, C.G., Henney, V., King, G., Moore, D.C., Dzimitrowicz McManus, H., Anderson, H.M., Moriarty, K.A., Di Valerio Gibbs, K. and Morgan, R.L. (2025) ONS/ASCO guideline on the management of antineoplastic extravasation. *JCO Oncology Practice*, 22(6) 1–15, OP-25-00579 DOI:10.1200/OP-25-00579

West Midlands Cancer Alliance (WMCA 2024) Guidelines for the Management of Extravasation of a Systemic Anti-Cancer Therapy including Cytotoxic Agents, V3 2024 available at: https://wmcanceralliance.nhs.uk/professionals-area/expert-advisory-groups/systemic-anti-cancer-therapy-sact

CHAPTER 4

Informed Consent

Emma Filby

Introduction

This chapter explores the complex perception of 'informed consent' in relation to the administration of systemic anti-cancer therapy (SACT). It examines the importance and types of consent, together with the legislation and cancer-specific guidance that informs and governs practice when obtaining informed consent. The chapter also considers the challenges and ethical dilemmas faced when obtaining informed consent, including the longevity of consent and how to ensure consent obtained is properly informed through the provision of timely and appropriate person-centred information.

Informed Consent

Within healthcare, consent refers to the process of obtaining agreement from a patient before providing treatment or initiating a procedure (Department of Health and Social Care, 2009). According to the National Health Service (2022), "Consent to treatment means a person must give permission before they receive any type of medical treatment, test or examination". For consent to be valid, it must be obtained voluntarily, without coercion, and the person must have the cognitive ability to make the decision. Informed consent goes further than consent alone. It not only involves obtaining agreement to a procedure or treatment, but it also expects the person to fully understand the nature of the proposed intervention. For informed consent to be valid, the person must understand the benefits and risks of the proposed intervention and be aware of alternatives, if available (Thirumoorthy, 2023).

Historically, informed consent was not a prerequisite to procedures or treatments. Clinicians were legally required under the law (for example, under doctrines like battery or common assault) to obtain only what was known as "simple consent". This was to avoid potential litigation, rather than actively ensuring the patient had a full understanding (Criminal Justice Act, 1988; Kim, 2009; Bowman, Spicer and Iqbal,

 DOI: 10.4324/9781003516477-4

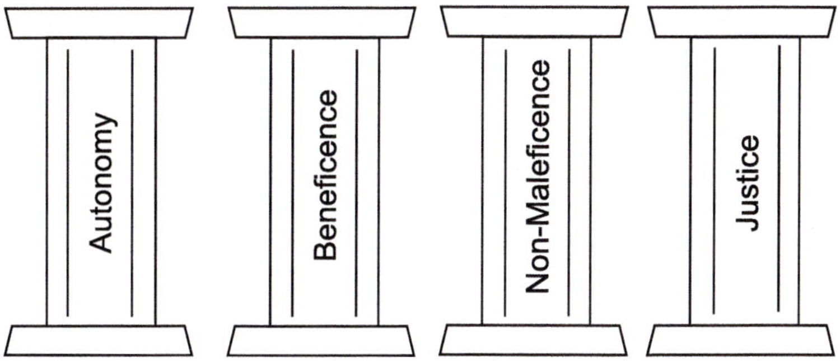

Figure 4.1 The Four Pillars of Medical Ethics

2012). However, legislation and healthcare practice have evolved substantially over time. Clinicians are now required to obtain informed consent before any intervention. Not only as a legal safeguard, but also to ensure principles like beneficence and non-maleficence (Figure 4.1), as mandated by professional regulators, such as the General Medical Council or Nursing and Midwifery Council.

It is considered that by providing the appropriate information about the intended outcomes and potential risks of proposed interventions, we are supporting patient understanding, thus promoting autonomous decisions. In principle, by promoting autonomous decisions, we can achieve valid informed consent. In today's healthcare landscape, where people are encouraged to make their own choices about their care and treatment, informed consent is imperative. For healthcare concordance, ensuring compliance with agreed interventions, there must be full involvement of the patient in the decision-making process, with all the necessary information to make informed choices and provide the required informed consent. In essence, no treatment or procedure should be attempted until the person receiving the intervention understands the implications of agreeing or declining the proposed options. Although informed consent sounds straightforward in principle, in practice it is complex and often poses legal and ethical challenges, which will be explored later in this chapter.

Types of Consent

Within healthcare, there are three main recognised forms of consent. These are verbal, written and implied, all of which play a role in the safe delivery of SACT. The United Kingdom Oncology Nursing Society (UKONS) SACT passport outlines the importance of ensuring patients are fully informed and actively consenting throughout their treatment journey, highlighting that consent is a process rather than a single one-off event at the beginning of treatment (UKONS, 2023).

Verbal Consent

Verbal consent is the most frequently used type of consent in clinical practice and occurs in day-to-day interactions. In the context of SACT, verbal consent is routinely obtained before each administration or cycle. For example, prior to the administration of SACT, the administering practitioner performs a toxicity screen to confirm the patient is well enough to proceed with treatment. At the same time, the administering practitioner obtains verbal confirmation from the patient that they are happy to proceed with the intended cycle of treatment. The verbal confirmation between the administering practitioner and patient allows the practitioner to assess the patient's understanding of treatment-related side effects and provides an opportunity to strengthen education around self-management. In general, this process serves to protect the patient from harm (NMC, 2018).

Assessing whether the patient is clinically well enough to receive treatment and confirming their continued willingness to proceed supports concordance with treatment, safe administration of SACT, and verifies that consent remains valid. Overall, the SACT administering practitioner confirms verbally with the patient's agreement to proceed with their treatment on that day. Although verbal consent is a less formal process than that of written consent, verbal consent plays a critical role in ongoing dialogue and supporting the principle that consent must be continuous and informed.

Written Consent

Consent is a legal and professional requirement before the commencement of any procedure or treatment. However, *written* consent is not considered a legal requirement; it is a formal record of evidence confirming that the consent process has taken place between the clinician and the patient. Therefore, protecting both the patient and clinician, demonstrating that the patient has been adequately informed of the intervention in line with legal standards, as set out in the Montgomery versus Lanarkshire UK Supreme Court judgment (2015). Written consent verifies confirmation that the patient has agreed to the proposed procedure or treatment at the time of discussion and the patient has been informed of the benefits, risks and alternatives. It does not, however, imply continued or unconditional agreement. In cancer, where treatments are complex, high-risk and often associated with significant toxicity, potentially impacting activities of daily living (Roper, Logan and Tierney, 2000), written consent is fundamental for transparency, accountability and governance. It is therefore important to note that written consent should not be viewed as a one-off signature, but a continual process, as part of a consent pathway, which supports safe, coordinated person-centred care.

The NCAG (2009) report promotes the use of standardised, treatment-specific written consent forms for SACT administration. This is to ensure that details regarding toxicities, risks and benefits are clearly documented and patients have been provided appropriate written information when consenting to treatment. The use of leaflets, videos and the pre-treatment consultations, delivered by a competent practitioner, supports the informed consent process by revisiting elements within the consent form, such as the risks, side effects and self-management advice. These processes not only strengthen the informed consent process, but also promote patient concordance, safety and person-centred coordinated care. Written consent should be obtained using either an organisationally approved SACT consent form or the national SACT regimen-specific consent forms (National Chemotherapy Board, 2016). It is the organisation's decision, following a strict governance process, on the type of form used, but essentially, the written consent form is signed by both the prescribing clinician and the patient.

Implied Consent

Implied consent is a less formal type of consent and is often inferred from a patient's actions or cooperation with a proposed intervention. For example, when a patient sits in a treatment chair and extends their arm to allow the practitioner to insert a venous access device for the intended SACT treatment. The action suggests agreement to proceed with the intervention. However, it is important to note that although implied consent is recognised as a form of consent, it does not replace verbal or written consent for SACT administration. Implied consent relies on body language, which can be easily misinterpreted, therefore, the validity of implied consent could be argued. Instead, based on the high-risk nature of SACT, implied consent acts to complement other forms of consent by reflecting ongoing patient willingness to engage with treatment. Practitioners delivering SACT must remain vigilant, as implied behaviours alone are not sufficient to demonstrate valid informed consent without prior verbal and written agreement.

Stop and Think

When and who should confirm consent?

Importance of Consent

SACT encompasses a wide range of treatments, inclusive of cytotoxic chemotherapy, targeted therapies and immunotherapies. Each therapy has varying levels of complexity and potential risk. These treatments carry significant toxicity profiles, which differ in severity (see Chapter 6). Due to these complexities, patients must be provided with personalised, clear, accurate, evidence-based information to promote autonomy when making treatment decisions. It is essential to ensure patients fully understand both the expected benefits and the potential adverse outcomes. The high-risk nature of SACT necessitates careful attention when obtaining informed consent, as it is the foundation of patient safety, professional accountability and ethical practice.

From a nursing perspective, the Nursing and Midwifery Council (NMC) Code (2018) emphasises that practitioners must act in the best interests of the patient, provide appropriate information to enable informed decision-making and respect the autonomy of the patient throughout their care. SACT practitioners are responsible for ensuring patients understand the nature of their treatment, anticipated side effects and treatment

Table 4.1 Consent and the NMC Code

Prioritise People	*Preserve Safety*	*Practice Effectively*	*Promote Professionalism and Trust*
Acting in the best interests of the patient Respecting the patient's autonomy	Reduce risk through understanding and clarification	Providing information to support informed decision-making	Ongoing consent across repeated treatment cycles

management, especially during repeated cycles of therapy, where treatment plans may alter due to toxicity or disease progression. This reinforces the principle of informed consent being a continuous process, not a single event. Therefore, it is important to understand the significance of SACT practitioners and the crucial role in assessing patients' understanding, clarifying information and providing education. These actions align with the NMC standards but importantly support patients to make autonomous decisions. Table 4.1 illustrates how these actions directly relate to the NMC (2018) Code and its priorities and demonstrates how SACT practitioners align with the NMC Code when ensuring consent before treatment.

Valid informed consent in SACT requires a balance of both verbal discussion and written documentation. Verbal discussion should facilitate the shared decision-making process leading to concordance, but also support the exploration of a patient's beliefs and values. As a result, this will assist in the monitoring of therapy side effects and self-management strategies. Written documentation, on the other hand, provides the important legal record of the initial agreement, offering protection for both the patient and the SACT healthcare team (GMC, 2020; NHS, 2022).

Challenges to Obtaining Informed Consent

Due to the nature of SACT administration, the cycle approach can present some challenges in obtaining continuous consent. This is based on the treatment modifications which can occur due to therapy toxicity or disease progression. Consequently, practitioners must revisit consent at each cycle or stage, ensuring patients remain informed and able to make autonomous, informed decisions. Recognising consent as a dynamic process

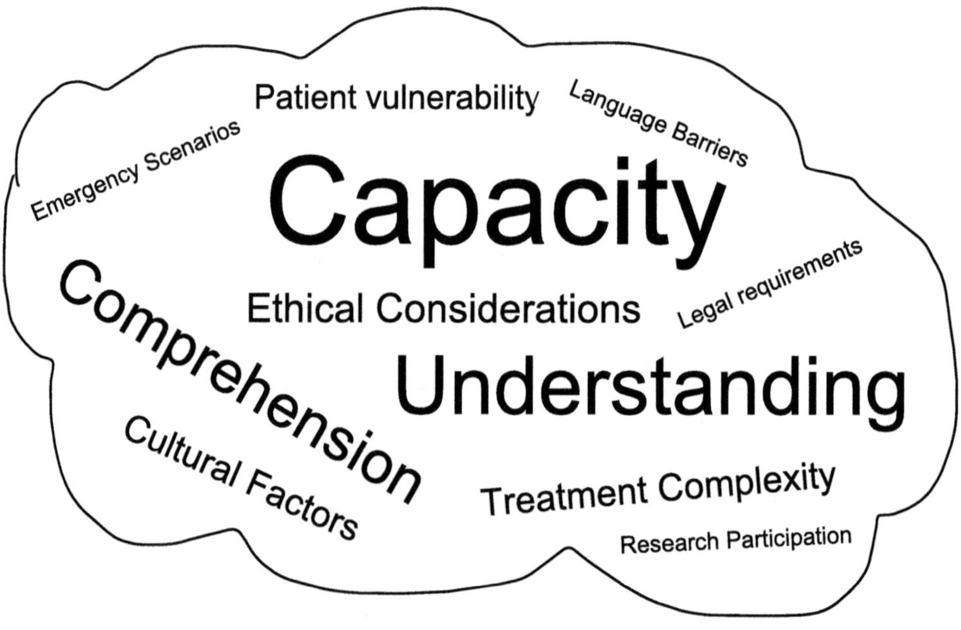

Figure 4.2 Word cloud highlighting challenges

enhances patient autonomy, promotes concordance with treatment and ensures SACT practitioners align with ethical, legal and professional obligations. There are multiple factors which influence the ability to obtain informed consent for SACT treatment (Figure 4.2).

Factors such as capacity, ethical considerations, legal requirements and treatment complexity. SACT practitioners play a key role in navigating these challenges.

Mental Capacity

Under the Mental Capacity Act (2005), adults are presumed to have decision-making capacity unless proven otherwise. The easiest way to identify if a patient has capacity is if the patient can understand, retain, consider information, and communicate a decision. If one of these elements is missing, capacity could be questionable.

Cancer patients may experience temporary cognitive impairment due to fatigue or emotional distress caused by the disease or treatment side effects. However, there are other chronic cognitive impairments which can affect a person's capacity, such as long-term health conditions like dementia, learning disabilities, brain injury, cerebral vascular accident (CVA) and mental health conditions, like depression and bipolar disorder. These factors, whether temporary or long term can pose challenges in obtaining informed consent. Although temporary cognitive impairments are, as the term suggests, transient, they must be taken into consideration when obtaining informed consent. Therefore, when capacity is questionable, concerns must be escalated following the appropriate processes, to ensure patient safety and advocacy, but also protect clinicians based on the ethical and legal principles surrounding informed consent.

Research and Clinical Trials

SACT can involve participation in clinical trials, including randomised, blind or double-blind studies. Intentions to join a clinical trial can pose complexities around obtaining informed consent. Patients participating in clinical trials must be briefed and understand the trial objectives, randomised trial processes, including the possibility that they may receive a placebo, but they will not know. This information is not in place of, but in addition to standard SACT treatment information. Before consent can be obtained, the designated consenting practitioner for the clinical trial must ensure the patient has a full understanding of the risks and benefits of the trial, to ensure valid informed consent. There are stringent protocols to follow with informed consent for clinical trials, including structured discussions, standardised documentation and a process for verification of patient understanding.

Administering SACT practitioners must also ensure ongoing informed consent throughout treatment delivery. Any administering practitioner must be familiar with the clinical trial objectives and the processes, especially as any treatment protocols evolve, or new evidence emerges during the study. Therefore, SACT practitioners must keep up to date on their clinical trial when involved in the administration of trial regimens. This ensures the practitioner remains in line with drug administration policies and guidelines, and enables them to convey accurate information to patients, to facilitate ongoing, valid informed consent.

Emergency Consent

There are some exceptions within medicine, when treatment can be delivered without consent. Consent may not be necessary if the emergency treatment is to preserve life or if the person is unconscious. However, if the person survives, a full explanation must be given to the person explaining why the treatment was necessary. Consider this as an example, a patient is admitted to an Intensive Care Unit (ICU) with advanced Acute Myeloid Leukaemia (AML), the patient is unconscious and deteriorating and requires an emergency administration of SACT to save their life. As they are unconscious, they are unable to consent. However, without treatment, the patient will die. Therefore, there are stringent processes in place within each organisation, heavily associated with governance and legal teams, to support clinicians with the decision-making process on treatment. There are, of course, complexities within the decision-making process, including family involvement, but ultimately, the healthcare professionals follow policy and ethical law to guide decisions in an emergency, to ensure that the best interests of the patient are being considered.

Speed of Diagnosis

Due to the importance of detecting cancer early to increase survival (Department of Health and Social Care, 2026), a person can receive a diagnosis of cancer with some degree of speed. This speed can influence a person's emotional state, understanding or ability to make informed decisions. This could be placed within the category of temporary cognitive impairment, as discussed earlier within mental capacity. Temporary cognitive impairment aside, the sense of urgency in deciding between treatment options can cause stress and anxiety. This may lead to decisions to decline treatment, with reasons relating to personal circumstances, like holidays, personal commitments or work. A person is absolutely entitled to decline treatment, but it is then questionable that the person is fully informed enough to decide, let alone provide informed consent. This behaviour could be an internal response to maintain control over what is life-changing.

The speed of diagnosis and consent can also impact a person when they are first given a diagnosis, where a diagnosis consultation feels like a distant memory. The person may agree to treatment and sign a consent form but leave with only the words "you have cancer" and a handful of leaflets. The prognosis, the treatment options, risks and benefits are lost to the ether, raising the question of obtaining "informed consent", once again highlighting the importance of consent being a continual process. Once a patient is given a diagnosis, patients are assigned a key worker, normally a clinical nurse specialist (CNS) and is given the opportunity to attend a pre-treatment consultation. This is intended to support the patient emotionally but also provide information supporting the informed consent process.

Responsibility and Accountability

In short, obtaining valid informed consent is everyone's business, much like the notion within Acute Oncology. Patients follow an individualised cancer pathway, designed to support person-centred care and as a result, many healthcare professionals are involved in the SACT pathway to ensure care is coordinated and responsive to patient need.

Therefore, it is not the responsibility of a single healthcare professional to obtain informed consent, it is the collective responsibility across the cancer multidisciplinary team. While responsibility is shared, accountability is distinct. Accountability safeguards both the patient and the practitioner by ensuring that informed consent meets legal, ethical and organisational requirements. This accountability sits with the designated healthcare professionals at specific points along the SACT pathway. Each practitioner involved in a patient's cancer pathway has a responsibility to support the informed element of consent, regardless of role. For example, a research nurse may explain the components of a clinical trial, while a SACT practitioner undertakes pre-treatment consultation. All contribute to ensuring the patient is informed. However, consent itself must be formally obtained by the appropriate clinician before proceeding with cancer-related treatment or procedures.

When considering accountability, certain roles carry specific responsibility for ensuring compliance with legal and professional standards. The clinician obtaining the written informed consent must ensure that the patient has been fully informed of the risks, benefits and alternatives to treatment. Similarly, the SACT practitioner responsible for treatment administration must confirm that all pre-treatment checks are complete, valid consent is in place and the patient remains informed and willing to proceed, including gaining final verbal consent prior to administration. Failure to meet these standards poses risks to both patient safety and professional practice. It may result in breaches of key ethical principles, including beneficence and non-maleficence, as well as non-compliance with the NMC (2018) Code.

Stop and Think

Who is responsible for gaining consent?

Longevity of Consent

The longevity of consent varies and depends on the circumstances. UK GDPR (Information Commissioner's Office, 2026) stipulate that there is no defined expiry timeframe for consent. However, it may no longer remain valid over time depending on changes in context. When considering the complexities of cancer, there are many important factors to evaluate, including prognosis, staging, disease behaviour, treatment options, treatment availability and potential side effects. These factors create multiple points within the patient pathway where consent may need to be reviewed and where appropriate, renewed. For example, if a patient's disease progresses on their current treatment and a second-line treatment is available, further informed consent would be required. This would typically involve a new written consent process and a further pre-treatment consultation to ensure consent remains valid and informed.

In addition to the evolving nature of cancer care, patients retain the right to withdraw consent at any time. A patient's decision may change based on their beliefs, values and perceptions of treatment, including the impact of side effects, or disease progression. As previously discussed, consent is an ongoing process, not a single event. Every individual has the right to revoke consent and discontinue treatment or procedures at any stage. These decisions must be respected, even where they do not align with medical advice, family wishes or personal views of healthcare professionals. This is particularly important when considering the longevity of consent, as a patient's decision may change over time. This reinforces the importance of the "informed" aspect of consent, recognising that consent must remain valid throughout the patient pathway, not just at the point it is initially obtained. Consent must therefore be obtained in line with professional standards, ensuring patients are fully informed and free from coercion, as outlined by the NMC (2018). As healthcare professionals, it is vital to remain non-judgmental and to respect the decisions of patients who have the capacity to make them, especially where those decisions can evolve. This includes ensuring that patients are provided with clear, evidence-based information at each stage of the pathway to support ongoing, informed decision-making.

Stop and Think

How long does consent last?

Patient Information

As alluded to throughout this chapter, information is key to enabling individuals to make informed decisions and therefore, provide informed consent. How that information is delivered varies across the healthcare system. Within SACT delivery, a substantial amount of complex information must often be conveyed within a relatively short timeframe. The information must be comprehensible, relevant and tailored to the individual, reflecting the principles of person-centred care. As aforementioned, it should include the benefits, risks, alternatives and potential side effects of treatment.

There are several key documents which guide practice and organisational policy in relation to SACT information delivery, making recommendations on how and when information should be shared with patients (Table 4.2).

While approaches to information provision vary across organisations, services are expected to align with national recommendations to meet agreed standards. These standards promote patient safety, consistency of practice, treatment concordance, and equity of access across cancer care. In essence, information provision should be coordinated, person-centred and integrated throughout the patient pathway. As with consent, information provision is an ongoing process rather than a one-off event. Information must be timely, clear and free from unnecessary jargon, delivered by the appropriate healthcare professional using a range of approaches. This may include physical written leaflets, videos, face-to-face discussions, or group sessions, using verbal, written and digital formats. It should be delivered in advance, wherever possible, allowing patients time to reflect and ask questions, while remaining focused to avoid information overload. Striking the right balance before SACT administration can be quite challenging. The volume and complexity of information, combined with time constraints, create a risk of information saturation. Patients may receive large amounts of information in multiple formats, which can affect their ability to process and retain key details. This is even more important as patients are often already feeling overwhelmed following a cancer diagnosis, navigating multiple appointments and facing emotional distress. At such a critical moment, they are expected to make treatment decisions, comply with

Table 4.2 National documents outlining information provision

Document	*Author/Year*	*Recommendations for the provision of information*	*Information provision timeline*
For Better, For Worse?	NCEPOD (2008)	• Support decision-making process • Consistent processes • Avoid adhoc information provision sessions • Support informed consent, not confirm a premade decision • Use a range of formats • Information provision clearly documented	• Before treatment • Not retrospectively delivered
Chemotherapy Services in England: Ensuring Quality and Safety	National Chemotherapy Advisory Group (2009)	• Standardised approach to SACT information provision • Use of national consent forms and written materials • Embed information provision into formal care pathways and governance processes	• Before treatment • Allow patient reflection time and provide the ability to ask questions
Guidance on Consent for SACT	UK SACT Board/ Cancer Research UK (2016) Updated 2025	• Information provision should be a continued process, not a one-off event • Face to face discussion accompanied by national written consent documentation • Tailor and simplify information • Discourage same day consent	• Before treatment • Not on the day of treatment, unless no alternative • Allow patient reflection time
Patient Experience in Adult NHS Services (CG138)	NICE (2012) updated 2021	• Personalised information • Check patient understanding • Avoid overload • Use a range of formats • Joint decision-making	• At key decision points throughout care pathways
Patient Experience in Adult NHS Services (QS15)	NICE (2012)	• Clear and consistent information • Patient involvement • Relate to patient experience	• Ongoing throughout care pathways
Shared Decision Making Guidance	NICE (2021)	• Supports shared decision-making • Decision-making aids • Structured conversations • Provide options	• Before care or treatment decisions
National Cancer Plan for England	Department of Health and Social Care and NHS England (2026)	• Consistency, equity of access • Multiple formats (inclusive of digital)	• Across the cancer pathway • Emphasis on timely provision

instructions for side effect management and be reassured that the decision remains theirs. It is therefore imperative that information is provided carefully and compassionately.

Recognising the potential impact of poor quality or excessive information on decision-making, it is essential to monitor both the quality of information provided and the support patients feel they receive. This enables organisations to measure their performance against national standards, with a focus on service enhancement, improved patient experience and supporting equity across the healthcare system. Ultimately, this supports a more informed decision-making process and a more robust consent process. The NHS England (2026) National Cancer Patient Experience Survey supports this approach, asking patients directly to share their experiences across the cancer pathway, specifically assessing whether they felt adequately informed and supported at key stages of their SACT journey.

Summary

In summary, informed consent is a mandatory requirement of SACT administration. Consent, regardless of its type, must be obtained by the appropriate practitioner and clearly documented in accordance with organisational policy. While there are recognised challenges in obtaining genuine informed consent, due diligence is required to ensure that consent is accurate, valid and meaningful. Consent has no official date of expiration, meaning consent must be a continuing process and can be withdrawn at any point by the patient. It is therefore imperative that consent is clearly and accurately documented for the safety of both the patient and the practitioner.

Facilitating informed consent is a shared multi-disciplinary responsibility. However, the accountability for obtaining consent rests ultimately with the practitioner undertaking the procedure or administering the treatment. Education is paramount in this process and healthcare professionals must ensure that information is provided in a timely, appropriate and compassionate manner to support patient understanding, confidence in decision-making and clarity in their decision for consent, therefore promoting concordance.

References

Bowman, D., Spicer, J. and Iqbal, R. (2012) *Informed consent: A primer for clinical practice.* 1st edition. Cambridge: Cambridge University Press.

Criminal Justice Act 1988 (c.33). UK Public General Acts. London: HMSO. Available at: www.legislation.gov.uk/ukpga/1988/33/content

Department of Health and Social Care (2009) *Reference guide to consent for examination or treatment.* 2nd edition. GOV.UK, London.

Department of Health and Social Care and NHS England (2026) *The National Cancer Plan for England: Delivering world class cancer care.* GOV.UK, London.

General Medical Council (2020) Decision making and consent. Accessed on 05 September 2025. [online] at: www.gmc-uk.org/professional-standards/the-professional-standards/decision-making-and-consent

Information Commissioner's Office (2026) What is valid consent? Accessed on 06 January 2026. [online] at: https://ico.org.uk/for-organisations/uk-gdpr-guidance-and-resources/lawful-basis/consent/what-is-valid-consent/#

Kim, S.Y.M. (2009) *Evaluation of capacity to consent to treatment and research.* New York: Oxford Academic https://doi.org/10.1093/med:psych/9780195322958.003.0001

National Chemotherapy Advisory Group (2009) *Chemotherapy services in England: Ensuring quality and safety*. London: National Chemotherapy Advisory Group.
National Chemotherapy Board (2016) Consent for Systemic Anti-Cancer Therapy (SACT). Accessed on 06 January 2026 [online] at: https://www.cancerresearchuk.org/health-professional/treatment-and-other-post-diagnosis-issues/consent-forms-for-sact-systemic-anti-cancer-therapy
National Confidential Enquiry into Patient Outcome and Death (2008) *For better, for worse? A review of the care of patients who died within 30 days of receiving systemic anti-cancer therapy*. London: National Confidential Enquiry into Patient Outcome and Death.
National Institute for Health and Care Excellence (2021) *Patient experience in adult NHS services: Improving the experience of care for people using adult NHS services (CG138)*. London: National Institute for Health and Care Excellence. Available at: www.nice.org.uk/guidance/cg138
National Institute for Health and Care Excellence (2012) Patient experience in adult NHS services (QS15). London: NICE. Updated 2019. Available at: www.nice.org.uk/guidance/qs15
National Institute for Health and Care Excellence (2021) Shared decision making (NG197). London: NICE. Available at: www.nice.org.uk/guidance/ng197
National Health Service (2022) Consent to treatment. Accessed on 05 Sep 2025. [online] at: www.nhs.uk/tests-and-treatments/consent-to-treatment/
NHS England (2026) About the survey. Accessed 06 January 2026 [online] at: https://www.cancerresearchuk.org/health-professional/treatment-and-other-post-diagnosis-issues/consent-forms-for-sact-systemic-anti-cancer-therapy
NMC (2018) *The code: Professional standards of practice and behaviour for nurses, midwives and nursing associates*. London: NMC.
Roper, N., Logan, W. and Tierney, A.J. (2000). *The Roper-Logan-Tierney model of nursing: Based on activities of living*. London: Churchill Livingstone.
Thirumoorthy, T. (2023) Core concepts of consent in medical practice. *Singapore Medical Journal*, 64(6), pp. 398–402 doi: 10.4103/singaporemedj.SMJ-2023-044.
UK Systemic Anti-Cancer Therapy Board (2025) *Guidance on Consent for Systemic Anti-Cancer Therapy (SACT)*. London: UK SACT Board and Cancer Research UK.
UKONS (2023) Systemic Anti-Cancer Therapy (SACT) competency passport. Accessed on 05 September 2025 [online] at: www.hee.nhs.uk/sites/default/files/documents/CapitalNurse%20SACT%20Passport%20framework.pdf

CHAPTER 5

Health and Safety

Alison Simons

Introduction

In this chapter, we will explore the occupational exposure risk of cytotoxic drugs and the routes of exposure. We will look at how to assess, monitor and reduce the risks and explain the current legislation and guidelines available. The hierarchy of control of risk and the use of hazardous drugs (HDs) safety measures will be discussed. The risk of exposure during the management of a cytotoxic spillage incident will be explored, including advice on how to minimise this risk of exposure during this procedure and the supportive guidelines available. Finally, the health and safety risks for patients and caregivers will be identified and the advice and information required will be discussed.

Occupational Exposure to SACT

HD (also now referred to as Hazardous Medicinal Products (HMP)) in the form of cytotoxic chemotherapy have been used to treat cancer for over half a century and today are used widely in a variety of healthcare settings and the community. Chapter 2 outlined the mechanism of action of cytotoxic chemotherapy, causing damage to DNA and thus inducing apoptosis of cells. Due to this action, some cytotoxic chemotherapy agents are categorised as hazardous substances as they may present hazards due to them being carcinogenic (cancer causing), mutagenic (cause mutations of DNA) reprotoxic (cause toxic effects on the reproductive system) and teratogenic (interferes with normal foetal development) (COSHH, 2002; Health and Safety Executive (HSE), 2017; NIOSH, 2024). These adverse effects are not only explicit to people receiving them therapeutically, but also to any personnel who may be exposed when handling them. Thus, accidental occupational exposure risks are present for any personnel who handle HD, and this means they could be exposed to this risk on a regular basis, over a long period of time (European Policy Recommendations Guidelines, 2019; European Biosafety Network, 2024).

DOI: 10.4324/9781003516477-5

Inhalation	Absorption	Digestion	Injection
When aerosols and drug particles are breathed in	When the drug is absorbed by the body via the skin and mucous membranes	When the drugs enter the digestive system	Accidental injection of drugs
• Reconstitution within the pharmacy aseptic unit. • Transport and storage • A splash or spillage incident, • Disposal of excreta of a patient who is receiving these drugs • Changing bed linen • Direct handling of the drugs such as drawing up and administration.	• Reconstitution within the pharmacy aseptic unit. • Transport and storage • A splash or spillage incident, • Disposal of excreta of a patient who is receiving these drugs • Changing bed linen • Direct handling of the drugs such as drawing up and administration.	• Poor hand hygiene, and then touching mouth, eyes etc. • Eating, drinking or smoking in a contaminated area • Poorly maintained sluice cleanliness	• Needle stick injury

Figure 5.1 Routes of exposure, how and when this may occur

Surface Contamination and Routes of Exposure

Due to potential droplet and aerosol formation, any surface can become contaminated with HD particles. Surface contamination and the risk of exposure to HDs can occur at any point along the journey of the drug, from preparation and reconstitution, transportation, storage, administration, patient and clinical waste disposal and if there is a splash or spillage of these drugs. The most common places to find contamination are on the nurse's station, sluice, other clinical areas, drip stands, the floor around the drip stands and patients' toilets (Eisenberg et al., 2021).

There are four main routes of accidental exposure to these drugs (HSE, 2017). Figure 5.1 outlines the routes of exposure and give some examples of how and when this exposure can occur.

Assessing, Controlling and Monitoring the Risk

The Health and Safety at Work Act (1974) is a piece of legislation covering occupational health and safety in Great Britain. It sets out the duties that the employer has towards employees and members of the public, employees have to themselves and to each other and the self-employed have towards themselves and others. This legislation is not explicit and is ambiguous using the term 'dangerous substances' or 'offensive substances' and this is because there was no official classification of specific substances, this came much later.

The Control of Substances Hazardous to Health (COSHH, 2002) regulations stipulates the legal requirements to control exposure to materials in the workplace that can make people ill. By the time of publication of this regulation, there was evidence that cytotoxic chemotherapy was hazardous, so was applicable to workplace settings which handled them. COSHH (2002) includes details of:

Assessing the risk to health

- Who might be harmed
- How workers may be exposed and the effected exposure by each of these routes
- How often people work with the substances and for how long
- Who else could be exposed such as maintenance workers, contractors and other visitors or members of the public

- What is already in place to control the risks
- What further action is needed to control the risks
- Who needs to carry out the action
- When is the action needed to be done by

Stop and Think ...

Answer the questions above and assess the risk for your clinical area.

Control the Risk and Protect Against Exposure

COSSH (2002) stipulates that the employer's overriding duty and priority is to consider how to prevent employees from being exposed to substances hazardous to health by all routes. Employees shall make full and proper use of any control measure, other thing or facility provided. The duty to prevent exposure should be achieved by measures other than the use of PPE. COSHH (2002) and HSE (2017) recommend using the principle of the hierarchy of control of risks of occupational exposure of HD (Figure 5.2). This principle aims to assist employers and employees in risk assessment and decision-making for workers handling these drugs. It is made up of five levels, starting with the most important and working down towards those ranked as less important.

(1) Elimination: This is the first consideration and suggests physically removing the hazard. This is not possible in the use of cytotoxic drugs as they are required to treat patients as part of their disease.
(2) Substitution: The second consideration is to replace the hazard, again this is not possible in terms of cytotoxic chemotherapy and if even one chemotherapy drug could be replaced it is more than likely replaced with another chemotherapy drug with similar hazards.

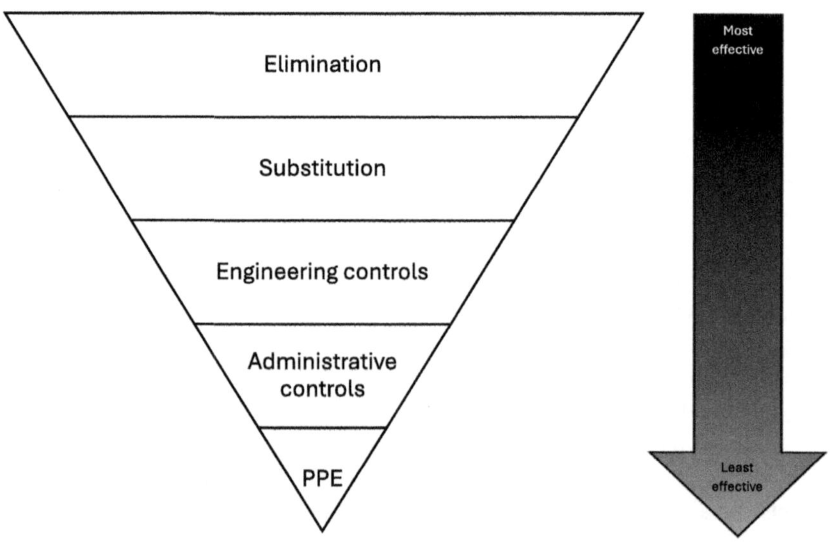

Figure 5.2 Hierarchy of controls

(3) Engineering controls: The next thing to consider is if people can be isolated from the hazard. Again, this is not possible as personnel are required to reconstitute, transport, store, administer and handle these drugs. However, the use of closed-system transfer devices (CSTD) could be considered in engineering controls in that they assist in minimising the risk of exposure to personnel by isolating the risk of the hazard being exposed.

(4) Administrative controls: The penultimate consideration is changing the way people work. Again, the use of CSTD should be considered here, to reduce the risk of exposure for all personnel handling these drugs including those who administer the drugs to patients. Other changes in working could also be explored for example the use of sealed clinical and patient waste equipment, procedures being employed to minimise risk of exposure, such as not spiking and not de-spiking infusion bags, not working above waist height, reviewing ventilation within clinical areas, and more emphasis on hand hygiene to mention a few. Training and education are key here.

(5) Personal Protective Equipment (PPE) is the final consideration and last resort if the proceeding layers cannot be implemented. This is to consider protection to the individual worker using equipment. Predominantly this is the use of aprons and gloves to handle these agents, however, the quality, suitability and availability of this equipment must also be contemplated. The use of full body gowns, armlets and gloves could be considered by employers, as these may provide more substantial protection than a thin apron that does not cover the workers' arms or clothing from potential exposure or contamination. Training and education on the correct use and scenarios of when to use PPE is recommended.

Inform, Instruct and Train About Risks and Precautions

COSHH (2002) states that every employer whose employees undertake work where there is a risk of exposure to hazardous substances must provide that employee with suitable and sufficient information, instruction and training. An overview of the key

Information

- Details and names of the substances hazardous to health
- Relevant workplace exposure or similar occupational
  •exposure limit
- Access to any relevant safety data sheet; and other legislative provisions which concern the hazardous properties of those substances
- Significant findings of the risk assessment

Training and Instruction

- Appropriate precautions and actions to be taken by the employee in order to safeguard himself and other employees at the workplace
- Results of any monitoring of exposure how and when to use the control measures;
- How to use PPE, and especially RPE, eg the correct method of removing and refitting gloves and masks, and determining how long protective gloves should be worn before any liquid contamination is liable to permeate them
- The cleaning, storage and disposal procedures they should follow, why they are required and when they are to be carried out,
- The risks of using contaminated PPE;
- The procedures to be followed in an emergenc

Figure 5.3 Key recommendations for information, training and instruction

recommendations are included in Figure 5.3. The information, instruction and training required must be provided in a manner appropriate to the level, type and duration of exposure identified, be ongoing and reviewed and updated whenever significant changes are made to the type of work carried out or to the work methods used.

Stop and Think …
Think about your training and instruction, did it meet these requirements?

Monitoring Exposure in the Workplace
COSHH (2002) and HSE (2017) recommends that monitoring is necessary where there is potential for exposure to carcinogenic compounds. As discussed earlier in Chapter 2 and this chapter, cytotoxic chemotherapy drugs are classified as carcinogenic. However, monitoring is only required if an occupational exposure limit or in-house working standard is in place to ensure these are not exceeded. There is currently no agreed safe limit of exposure to chemotherapy, so this makes it difficult to justify if monitoring of exposure should be undertaken. Other reasons monitoring may occur is if deterioration of control measures could result in a serious health effect or any change in the conditions affecting employee's exposure which could mean that adequate control is no longer being maintained. This is ambiguous and open to interpretation by each employer and organisation, and results in non-standardised approaches to monitoring and health surveillance for those handling HD.

Reducing Risk of Exposure/HD Safe Handling Measures
Several national and international documents have been published informing personnel of the safe handling measures required to reduce the risk of exposure to HD (European Policy Recommendations Guidelines, 2019, European Biosafety Network, 2024, ISOPP, 2022, NIOSH, 2024 European Agency for Safety and Health at Work (EU-OSHA, 2023). It is important to note that this guidance is more legally binding in some countries than others, and for some countries they are purely recommendations. In the main, these documents include information regarding safe handling measures for each point where there is risk.

Reconstitution
The raw concentrated agent needs to be manipulated to be used therapeutically; this is the point when there is the highest risk of surface contamination and occupational exposure. Therefore, reconstitution of HD takes place within the pharmacy aseptic environment or a specific compounding unit where strict regulations and specific equipment are mandatory. For example, reconstitution of these drugs must be performed in a controlled area with restricted access. The area must be well ventilated and designed to facilitate effective cleaning (ISOPP, 2022). Preparation of HD must take place within a biological safety cabinet (BSC) (see Figure 5.4). These are enclosed ventilated units designed to protect workers from exposure (in addition to reducing contamination), to hazardous

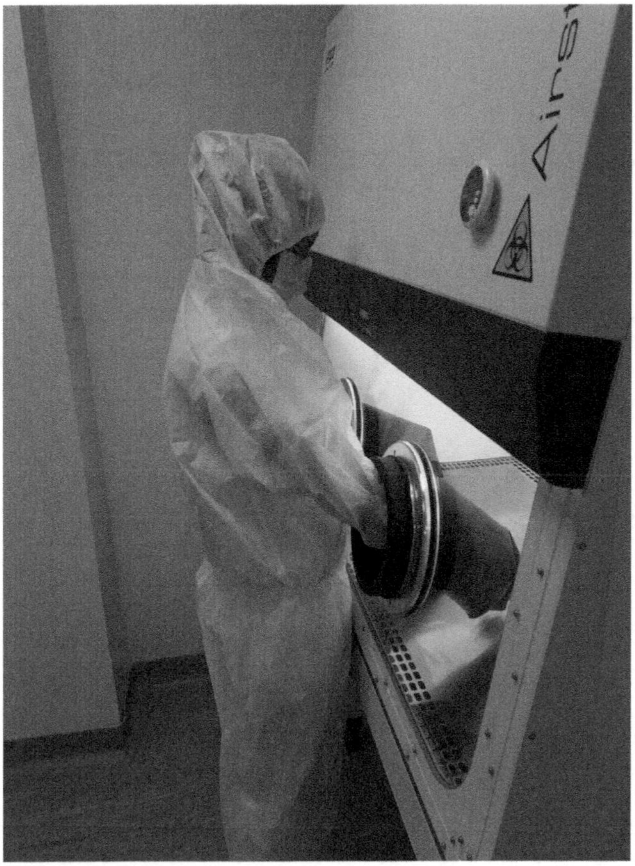

Figure 5.4 Biological safety cabinet in use

material by using airflow and filter systems (European Policy Recommendations Guidelines, 2019, European Biosafety Network, 2024, ISOPP, 2022, NIOSH, 2024, European Agency for Safety and Health at Work (EU-OSHA, 2023).

European Policy Recommendations Guidelines (2019), European Biosafety Network (2024), ISOPP (2022), NIOSH (2024) and European Agency for Safety and Health at Work (EU-OSHA) (2023) all state that within the BSC the use of closed system transfer devices (CSTD) must be used and acts as an additional level of protection. CSTD are devices that mechanically prohibit the escape of HD vapour concentrations outside of the system. In most countries, this is mandatory for reconstitution of these agents, they are optional for administration of these agents (see administration). Furthermore, extra quality control measures and regular physical monitoring of equipment are also required, such as pressure, particle counts, room air changes per hour, air velocity and filter integrity. The frequency of this monitoring varies across each measure, and can be required daily, monthly or annually. The highest level of PPE is required during reconstitution; the minimum must include protective gown/coveralls, protective gloves, protective face shield/goggles and respiratory protection.

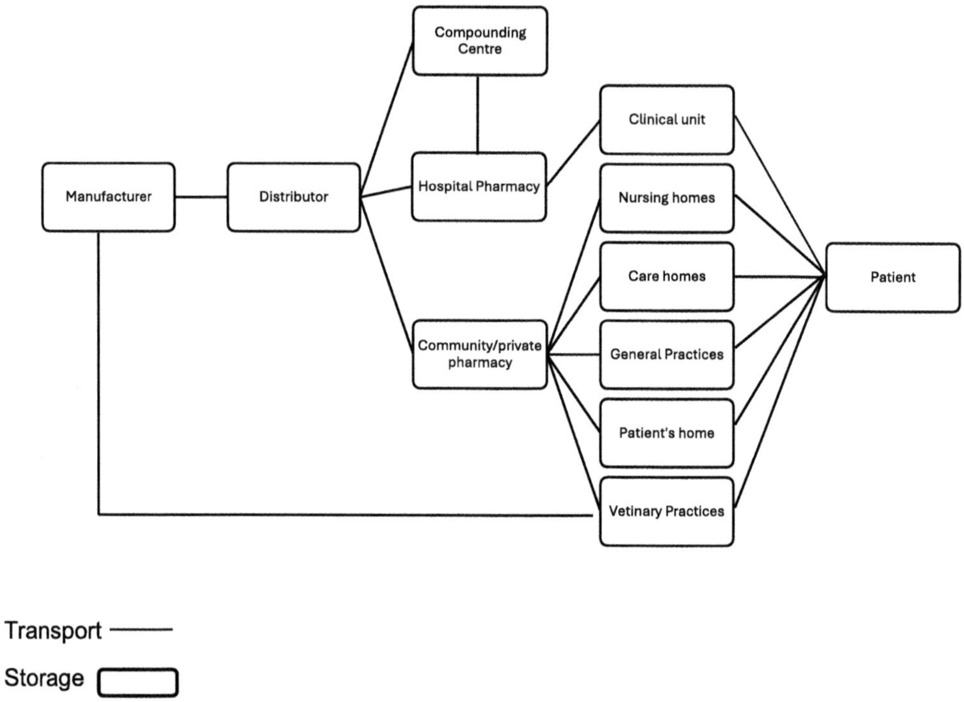

Figure 5.5 Transportation and storage

Transportation and Storage

HDs need to be transported and stored from and to a variety of locations. For example, the manufacturer will need to transport the drug to a distributor, who then transports them to pharmacies and compounding centres. Once reconstituted, they need to be transported to the administration site, which may be within the same or a different hospital. It could also be transported to veterinary practices or community settings such as nursing homes, care homes, general practices or patient's homes. At each location, HD safe storage policy needs to be adhered to, and between each location safe transportation needs to be undertaken. Figure 5.5 illustrates this roadmap and the numerous points at which the risk of exposure may occur. However, it does not show the journey of the drugs if they need to be returned, for example, due to expiration or quality concerns, which is an additional consideration (European Agency for Safety and Health at Work (EU-OSHA, 2023).

Packaging of HD

To facilitate safe transportation, packaging material must be selected based on its ability not to break, leak or spill. The use of plastic rather than glass where possible, and if not possible glass should be sealed in plastic leakproof wrappers. HD should be packaged separately from non HD. When packaging HD that have been reconstituted, they must be individually packed or sealed in secondary packing such as sealed plastic wrapping or container to prevent leakage or spillage. At the very minimum protective gloves should be worn during packaging HD and a spill kit should be easily available (see management of a spillage) (ISOPP, 2022, European Agency for Safety and Health at Work (EU-OSHA), 2023).

Labelling HD

HD must be clearly and easily identified to ensure all personnel are aware of the hazardous nature of the package. Many countries have a standard recognisable symbol indicating cytotoxic and/or hazardous substances, often with the words 'danger', 'caution' or 'hazard' clearly displayed. Additional information: the name of the agent, dosage date of preparation and expiry date should be included on the label (ISOPP, 2022, European Agency for Safety and Health at Work (EU-OSHA, 2023).

Administration of HD

HD are administered therapeutically in a variety of settings; HD can be administered in a variety of modes (see Chapter 10). Whilst previously acknowledged, handling the raw concentrated product is the highest risk of surface contamination and occupational exposure; this risk is strictly controlled and monitored. The risk of HD exposure during administration is still significant and the environments at risk of contamination widen. However, the risk is not subject to such rigorous control and monitoring. Guidelines and recommendations regarding safe handling including administration of HD are available but are not regulated or monitored for adherence in the main. Administration of HD must only be administered by personnel who have had adequate training and assessed as competent. Sadly training and competence is not currently consistent across areas that administer HD and the documents regarding training and competence are currently only recommendations in many places. The introduction of the SACT competency passport (UKONS) aims to address the inconsistency in SACT training within the United Kingdom. However, currently there has been no follow-up or evidence to support whether the aim of this intervention has been achieved and there is limited content within the passport regarding health and safety when handling HD. For reconstitution of HD in most countries, the use of CSTD is mandatory. However, they are only optional for the administration of these agents. More recently there has been a greater emphasis on using CSTD for the administration of HD, and in some countries it is now a requirement (European Biosafety Network, 2024 and United States Pharmacopeia (USP), 2020). This is not without opposition, such as compatibility of devices used in reconstitution and administration, microbiological contamination and the well-voiced concern that there is a potential additional cost associated with using these devices for administration. The latter argument can be offset in terms of the benefits of workers feeling valued and cared for, leading to motivation and contentment. This in turn results in a healthy workforce, reduced sickness rates and increased recruitment and retention of staff. Ultimately cost should not factor in an employer's legal responsibility to protect personnel from occupational exposure and risk of harm and life-changing impacts (European Biosafety Network, 2024) (see COSHH, 2002 and Health and Safety at Work Act, 1974).

A summary of the general principles for safe handling and administration of SACT are presented in Table 5.1.

Table 5.1 A summary of the general principles for safe handling and administration of SACT

Control of Exposure

- Use totally enclosed systems where reasonably practicable
- Do not de-spike empty infusion bags
- Control exposure at source, for example, by using adequate extraction systems and appropriate organisational measures
- Issue personal protective equipment where adequate control cannot be achieved by other measures alone
- Reducing the quantities of drugs used; the number of employees potentially exposed; and their duration of exposure, to the minimum
- Ensuring safe handling, storage and transport of cytotoxic drugs and waste material containing or contaminated by them
- Using good hygiene practices and providing suitable welfare facilities, for example prohibiting eating, drinking and smoking in areas where drugs are handled and providing washing facilities
- Training staff who handle cytotoxic drugs or deal with contaminated waste, on the risks and the precautions to take
- Provide annual updated training to all staff who handle SACT agents
- Make cleaning personnel aware of the risks of exposure to SACT agents and request they wear appropriate PPE when they work in SACT clinical areas

Personal Protective Equipment (PPE)

- PPE should be provided and used wherever risks cannot be adequately controlled in other ways
- PPE should be selected based on your risk assessment
- It is important that the PPE offers adequate protection for its intended use
- Employees must be trained in the use of PPE
- PPE must be adequately maintained and stored
- PPE should include:
- Chemotherapy gloves and gown, Eye/face Protection (if risk of emesis or splashes), Respiratory protection (if risk of inhalation)

Source: Adapted from NIOSH (2024), HSE (2017) and Santillo et al. (2018).

Spillage of HD

Risk and Management of HD Spillage

At any point during the handling of HDs there is risk of accidental spillage, and this can occur within a wide variety of environments. For example, during:

- Reconstitution process in pharmacy/aseptic unit
- Transportation to and from areas of manufacture, distribution and administration
- Storage in manufacture, reconstitution, transportation and administration settings
- Administration in clinical areas and patient's homes
- Disposal of patient and clinical waste
- Any area a patient may visit whilst receiving treatment (toilets, bathrooms, public areas)

This list is not exhaustive and illustrates the complexities involved in reducing, managing and monitoring risk of SACT spillage. The measures in place to reduce the risk of accidental exposure of HDs, as outlined in the previous sections, have the dual purpose of reducing the risk of spillage of these materials at each point on their journey. However, these do not encompass the considerations of patients wishing to walk around while receiving intravenous treatment. Although there should be robust measures in place to reduce the risk of spill incidents when handling HD, the risk cannot be eliminated.

Procedure for the Management of a Spillage of HD

All locations that work with HDs must have a spillage policy in place and a spillage kit that is easily accessible (European Biosafety Network, 2024). The content of the policy and kits will vary from place to place, so it is imperative that all personnel are familiar with the content and locations of policies and kits in the areas they are handling HDs.

Stop and Think ...

- What does your HD spillage policy include?
- Where is the spillage kit located in your clinical area?
- List the contents of your spillage kit.

The general principles of managing a HD spillage are typically to:

- Ask for assistance and for the spill kit
- Alert colleagues of spill
- Prioritise decontamination of anyone who has been exposed to HD (see Table 5.2)
- Prohibit people entering the area of the spill – put out signs to identify spillage area
- Mark the spill area
- Put on PPE as per policy and spill kit
- Prevent spill spreading and splashing
- Use drying/absorbent materials for liquids – use wet cloth for dry powders
- Work from outside to inside to clean up spill
- Remove all visible spill
- Clean contaminated area as per policy
- Rinse/dilute with water
- Dry area
- Repeat clean and dry actions at least three times
- Remove PPE
- Wash hands
- Dispose of all waste as per contaminated waste policy
- Inform colleagues when decontamination has been completed
- Complete required documentation

Table 5.2 outlines the general actions for managing personnel contamination.

Table 5.2 The general actions for managing personnel contamination

Contamination	*Actions*
Skin	Rinse exposed area with warm water, then wash thoroughly but not aggressively with neutral detergent, rinse skin with warm water, dry skin by dabbing but not rubbing. Seek medical advice
Eyes	Rinse eyes with suitable solution (warm water or saline) for 15 minutes using eye bath/shower. Seek medical advice
Clothes	Remove contaminated clothing as soon as possible. Treat clothing as per contaminated laundry policy: Wash separately and wash twice.
Needle stick injury	Follow needle stick injury policy. Seek medical advice

Source: European Biosafety Network, 2024.

Stop and Think ...

Describe the actions you would take if staff were contaminated by a SACT spillage that includes skin, eye and clothing contamination.

Documentation and Follow Up

Due to the implications of accidental exposure of HDs, it is imperative that any potential accidental exposure or spillage incident must be recorded. The purpose is to report the incident and provide documentation of what occurred, how and why. This serves as a safety alert and will identify any learning points from the incident that may require improvements in practices. It will also provide an evidence trail for the drug and why further HD reconstitution may be required. Ultimately it will provide important evidence of potential or actual exposure of HD for any individuals involved with the management of the spillage. It is advisable that this is also recorded on their personal occupational health record for future reference through an occupational health referral.

The documentation requirements may differ between institutions, but the following information should typically be recorded.

- Context of incident
- Date and location of incident
- Effected/exposed personnel
- HD involved
- HD concentrations if known
- Control measures employed

Stop and Think ...

- How would you replace your spillage kit once it has been used?
- What documentation would you complete after the spillage has been dealt with?
- Why is it important to document a spillage incident?

Training in Management of a HD Spillage

Employers have a responsibility to provide spillage training for those personnel who handle HD, regardless of their level of involvement. With the comprehensive measures that are in place to minimise the risk of a HD spill it should be a rare occurrence but as stated previously, unfortunately the risk cannot be eliminated. Due to the infrequency of such an incident, experience of how to manage a spill could be limited; personnel who have not experienced it may not have the skills, and those that have had experience may have forgotten. Familiarity with the contents of the spill kit and how to use the equipment may also be limited. Therefore, practical and simulated scenarios are recommended in spillage management training. This training should be delivered by personnel who are knowledgeable and competent in occupational health and safety, safe handling of HD and working environments. A particular focus should be on preventing personal exposure, other individuals' exposure and spreading contamination.

Patient and Caregiver Safety

As discussed earlier in this chapter the risk of exposure to HD is clear, however, this is not unique to healthcare personnel. Patients and their caregivers are also at risk of accidental exposure. Whilst there is legislation, guidance and recommendations on the safe handling of HD available for healthcare professionals, these are not specific or explicit in terms of the education required for patients and their caregivers. The risks and need for education are further compounded by the variety of settings in which SACT can be administered (see Chapter 10) with many patients receiving treatment in their own home. This means there is a risk of exposure from the HD being administered in that environment; this can sometimes be in the form of oral treatment administered by the patient or caregiver. There is also a risk of exposure from a patient's waste as HD can sometimes take up to 10 days to be excreted. It is worth noting that Cancer Research UK does provide this information on their website, but this is not general information and is not individualised to patients and their specific treatment or personal situation. Therefore, standardised and personalised patient and caregiver information is recommended to be developed and utilised for patients receiving SACT.

Advice for Safety at Home

Based on what we know in terms of the risks of exposure the following general information should be given to patients and caregivers as a minimum, and take-away written information is recommended (adapted from Cancer Research UK (2024)).

Patient Waste

- Close the lid and flush twice after using the toilet. To avoid splashing, men should urinate sitting down.
- Wash hands well with soap and water after using the toilet. Clean the area with soap and water if body fluids splashed on skin.
- Wear gloves when cleaning the toilet, wiping up bodily fluids such as urine, faeces, vomit, or changing incontinence pads. Wash hands with gloves on, remove them, and throw them in the household waste. Rewash hands.

- Clean the toilet daily with a product containing bleach.
- Carers should wear gloves when handling a bedpan or urinal. Empty the contents into the toilet close to the water. This will limit splashing. Keep the gloves on and wash the bedpan or urinal with soap and water after each use.
- Double bag incontinence pads and throw them in the household waste. For example, put the used pads in a bag or bin liner and then place this into another bin liner before throwing it in the household waste outside the home.
- Wear gloves when emptying the stoma bag. Wash the stoma bag daily with soap and water.

Handling Waste or Laundry

- Handle contaminated waste or laundry with gloves. Wash your hands before and after removing the gloves.
- Place contaminated waste in special bags if provided. Otherwise, double bag it in plastic, leakproof bags. Place in the regular household waste.
- For SACT via an ambulatory pump consider using a plastic mattress protector on the bed. This is to prevent chemotherapy spillage into the bed if an accident happens.
- If a spillage happens, wear gloves, blot the area dry with a kitchen towel, and remove the contaminated clothing or linen immediately.
- Wash the mattress or plastic mattress cover three times with warm, soapy water and let it dry.
- Wash soiled laundry straight away if possible. If you can't, place it in a leakproof plastic bag. Wash it as soon as possible.
- Wash soiled laundry separately from other laundry on the longest and hottest cycle. Wash twice without removing it from the machine between washes. Use regular laundry soap.
- Anyone who is pregnant, thinks they are pregnant, or who is breastfeeding should not handle contaminated waste or laundry. Wherever possible, they should ask someone else to do it.

Dealing with Spills

- Provide the patient with a spillage kit and instructions on how to use it.

Spills on Floors or Surfaces

- Always wear gloves to clean up.
- Alert others around you of the spill.
- Be careful not to step into the spill or get any on your shoes.
- Remove or turn off any fans in the direction of the spillage.
- Create a barrier with paper towels around the spillage so it doesn't spread further.
- Use paper towels to wipe up the spill.
- Clean the area with soap and water. Rinse the area using paper towels.
- Throw out waste in specially marked containers provided. Otherwise, double bag in leakproof plastic bags.
- Wash hands before and after removing gloves.

Spillage in the Eyes

- Wear gloves if you're a carer helping the person to wash their eyes.
- Wash the eyes with plenty of water for at least 10 minutes.
- Contact your advice line immediately or go to Accident and Emergency.
- Anyone who is pregnant, thinks they are pregnant, or who is breastfeeding should not deal with spills. Wherever possible, they should ask someone else to do it.

Contraception and Pregnancy

- Use barrier methods (condoms, femidoms or dental dams) during oral, vaginal or anal sex for as long as you've been advised to. This applies to both the patient and their partner.
- The patient and their partner should use effective birth control to prevent becoming pregnant while taking SACT. Depending on the drugs, this might be for several months or years after treatment. Some of these drugs can harm the developing baby (foetus), especially during weeks 1 to 12 (first trimester). Menstrual cycles can become irregular during and after treatment. So, it is not always possible to know if someone is at a time in their cycle when they could become pregnant or is pregnant.

Safety for Family and Friends

- It is safe to hug and kiss a partner, family or friends.
- It is safe to visit, sit with, hug, and kiss children.
- It is safe to be around pregnant women. But they should not clean up body fluids.
- It is safe to share a bathroom with others. If body fluids splash on the toilet, wear gloves and clean the area with soap and water. Others may use the toilet after it is cleaned it up.

SACT Tablets or Capsules at Home

- Keep tablets or capsules out of reach of children and pets.
- Always limit the handling of SACT tablets or capsules. Push them out from the packet into a small cup or pot, for example, a shot glass. Tip this into the mouth. If the patient is unable to do this, wash hands thoroughly with soap and water after handling these medicines. Keep the cup or pot separately for this purpose.
- Anyone helping with SACT tablets or capsules should wear gloves.
- Anyone who is pregnant, thinks they are pregnant, or who is breastfeeding shouldn't touch chemotherapy or hormone therapy tablets or capsules. If they must help, they should take extra care, wear disposable gloves, and tip them into a medicine cup.
- Never crush or chew these tablets or capsules. Swallow them whole. Contact advice line or speak to pharmacist if unable to do this.
- Some people may be directed by their pharmacist to crush tablets or open capsules. For example, if receiving medicines through a feeding tube. Follow the directions from the pharmacist on how to do this safely.

- Do not take another dose if vomiting occurs after taking SACT tablets or capsules. Contact advice line.
- Make sure course of treatment and the prescription is understood and how many tablets or capsules to take is clarified.
- Return unused tablets or capsules to the pharmacist at the hospital. Never flush any tablets or capsules down the toilet or throw them in the household waste.
- Contact advice line if too many tablets or capsules are taken by mistake.

Practical Things to Remember

- Throw empty SACT tablets or capsule bottles and boxes in the household waste (not the recycling).
- Return full or partly used bottles of SACT tablets, capsules or injections to the pharmacist at the hospital.
- Always wash hands thoroughly before and after handling SACT medicine or any spillage.
- Carers or family members should always wear disposable gloves if likely to encounter SACT.
- Change gloves immediately if they are torn or contaminated.
- Put used gloves into a bag and throw them in the household waste.

Stop and Think ...

What information do you provide to patients and caregivers who are receiving SACT at home or are discharged home following SACT?
Is this standardised information?
Is this person-centred information?
Do you support this with written information?

Summary

Cytotoxic chemotherapy agents are classified as HDs as they pose significant risk to health; the risk of accidental exposure is real. Employers have the legal responsibility to prevent employees from being exposed to substances hazardous to health by all routes, and that employees must make full and proper use of any control measures in place, other things or facilities provided. The legislation, policy, guidelines and recommendations on safe handling measures should be adhered to by all personnel handling HD, to ensure best and safe practice for themselves, other colleagues and the public. All personnel must be vigilant in terms of the hierarchy of controls, education and training. It is important to remember that the risk of exposure can occur at any point within the life cycle of the drug from reconstitution to disposal of patient's waste, and that HD can be handled in a wide variety of settings. Patients and caregivers are also at risk of accidental exposure, and we have a duty of care to inform them of the risks and provide information on how to mitigate these.

On a final note, the use of other therapies such as immunotherapies and biological therapies has significantly increased over recent years and as research advances it is likely that many other therapies will be discovered and drugs developed to treat cancer. Currently there is no data on the risk to health for personnel accidentally exposed to these agents and they are not classified as HD. It is worth considering that we do know how these drugs work on a cellular level (see Chapter 8) and although no risk has yet been identified this does not mean there is no risk and the consideration of safe handling measures may be wise.

References

Control of Substances Hazardous to Health Regulations (2002) Available at: www.legislation.gov.uk/uksi/2002/2677/contents

Eisenberg, S. et al. (2021) Hazardous drug contamination: Presence of bathroom contamination in an ambulatory cancer center. *Clinical Journal of Oncology Nursing*. [Online] 25(2), pp. 151–156.

European Agency for Safety and Health at work (2023) Guidance for the safe management of hazardous medicinal products at work. Available at https://osha.europa.eu/en/publications/guidance-safe-management-hazardous-medicinal-products-work

European Biosafety Network (2024) Preventing contamination, exposure and health impacts for workers from hazardous medicinal products (HMPs) at work by the implementation of closed systems in their manufacture and use. Available at: www.europeanbiosafetynetwork.eu/wp-content/uploads/2024/04/EBN-white-paper-on-HMPs__5.04.2024.pdf

European Policy Recommendations (2019). Preventing occupational exposure to cytotoxic and other hazardous drugs. Available at: www.europeanbiosafetynetwork.eu/wp-content/uploads/2016/05/Exposure-to-Cytotoxic-Drugs_Recommendation_DINA4_10-03-16.pdf

Cancer Research Uk (2024) Chemotherapy safety at home. Available at: www.cancerresearchuk.org/about-cancer/treatment/chemotherapy/chemotherapy-safety-at-home

Health and Safety at Work Act (1974) Available at: www.legislation.gov.uk/ukpga/1974/37/contents

Health and Safety Executive, (2017). Safe handling of cytotoxic drugs in the workplace. [online] Available at: www.hse.gov.uk/healthservices/safe-use-cytotoxic-drugs.htm

International Society of Oncology Pharmacy Practitioners (ISOPP), (2022) "ISOPP standards for the safe handling of cytotoxics." *Journal of Oncology Pharmacy Practice (England)* 28, no. 3_suppl (2022): S1. https://doi.org/10.1177/10781552211070933

National Institute for Occupational Safety and Health (2004). Preventing occupational exposure to antineoplastic and other hazardous drugs in health care settings. Available at www.cdc.gov/niosh/docket/archive/pdfs/NIOSH-105/0105-090104-alert.pdf

National Institute for Occupational Safety and Health (2016) NIOSH List of Antineoplastic and Other Hazardous Drugs in Healthcare Settings, 2016. www.cdc.gov/niosh/docs/2025-103/pdfs/2025-103.pdf?id=10.26616/NIOSHPUB2025103

Santillo, M., Field, A., Henderson, J. et al. (2018) Guidance on Handling of Injectable Cytotoxic Drugs in Clinical Areas in NHS Hospitals in the UK. www.sps.nhs.uk/wp-content/uploads/2018/07/Guidance-on-Handling-Cytotoxics-Ed-1-July-2018.pdf

United States Pharmacopeia (2020). *General chapter, ⟨800⟩ hazardous drugs—Handling in healthcare settings*. USP-NF. Rockville, MD: United States Pharmacopeia.

CHAPTER 6

Preparation and Monitoring of Patients Receiving SACT

Emma Filby

Introduction

There are many side effects associated with different systemic anti-cancer therapy (SACT) regimens. However, some side effects are more commonly anticipated across SACT treatments. Patients must be informed of these, and baseline measurements must be recorded before treatment commences. Each patient may experience side effects differently, in both type and severity. It is a little like a card game, not knowing the hand you will be dealt. This highlights that side effects are individual and can vary significantly from person to person, reinforcing the importance of personalised care planning. Patients often develop recognisable patterns of side effects across treatment cycles, enabling SACT practitioners to take a more proactive approach in supporting self-management and anticipating the potential need for further intervention or escalation. Therefore, structured preparatory assessment, monitoring and timely management are vital for both patient safety and treatment efficacy.

SACT Side Effects

Side effects are unpredictable in type and severity, as SACT works by targeting rapidly dividing cells to damage and destroy cancer cells (see Chapter 2). However, in doing so, it can also affect healthy cells that divide quickly, leading to temporary damage across different body systems. Many of these common side effects are short-term and usually improve or resolve once treatment has finished.

Stop and Think ...
Describe why cytotoxic chemotherapy affects healthy cells.

DOI: 10.4324/9781003516477-6

Factors Influencing Side Effects

Additional factors can influence the type and severity of side effects experienced. With increasing age physiological functions naturally decline, including renal, cardiac and pulmonary functions, which can affect treatment tolerance and increase susceptibility to side effects. In addition, the presence of existing comorbidities may further influence how well treatment is tolerated, while a patient's performance status also plays an important role in determining overall ability to cope with treatment and potential side effects. The ECOG performance status is used widely to support treatment decision-making, as it assesses a patient's level of functioning and helps determine whether they are fit enough to tolerate treatment. Table 6.1 outlines the ECOG Performance Status Scale.

Recognition of these influencing factors allows healthcare professionals to anticipate potential side effects and implement appropriate management strategies. These may include prophylactic pharmacological and non-pharmacological interventions, dose modifications and good patient education to support self-management. Table 6.2 outlines key influencing factors and potential management strategies.

Table 6.1 ECOG Performance Status Scale

Grade	*ECOG Performance Status*
0	Fully active, able to carry on all pre-disease performance without restriction
1	Restricted in physically strenuous activity but ambulatory and able to carry out work of a light or sedentary nature, e.g., light housework, office work
2	Ambulatory and capable of all self care but unable to carry out any work activities; up and about more than 50% of waking hours
3	Capable of only limited self care; confined to bed or chair more than 50% of waking hours
4	Completely disabled; cannot carry on any self care; totally confined to bed or chair
5	Dead

Source: Oken MM, Creech RH, Tormey DC, Horton J, Davis TE, McFadden ET, Carbone PP. Toxicity and response criteria of the Eastern Cooperative Oncology Group. *Am J Clin Oncol.* 1982 Dec;5(6):649-655. PMID: 7165009.

Credit: The ECOG Performance Status Scale was developed by the Eastern Cooperative Oncology Group (ECOG), now the ECOG-ACRIN Cancer Research Group, and published in 1982. To learn more, visit ecog-acrin.org/scale.

Table 6.2 Factors influencing side effects and potential management strategies

Factor category	*Examples of influencing factors*	*Management strategies*
Patient Factors	Age Comorbidities Performance Status	SACT dose modification SACT treatment delays Prophylactic medications (antiemetics, growth factors) Patient education Self-management strategies
Treatment Factors	Drug Dose Schedule Combination Therapy	

Patient Preparation for SACT

Preparatory Investigations

Preparing the patient before SACT is essential to ensure treatment is delivered safely. Preparatory investigations such as blood tests, organ function and other basic measurements (for example, blood pressure and weight) provide a baseline for comparison as the patient progresses through treatment. Establishing these baselines helps us understand what is "normal" for the patient, while also highlighting any areas that may require closer monitoring if there is an increased risk of side effects. This approach supports early identification of toxicity and helps maintain patient safety throughout the treatment. Some preparatory investigations are drug-specific, with organisational treatment protocols outlining the required parameters. Others are undertaken across all SACT regimens as part of best practice and risk assessment.

Height and Weight

The patient's height and weight are measured before treatment and in some organisations, this is carried out by two healthcare professionals to improve accuracy and reduce the risk of human error. These measurements are required to calculate the patient's body surface area (BSA), which is commonly used to determine the appropriate dose of treatment. To calculate the BSA, the height needs to be measured in centimetres and the weight in kilograms. The height is then multiplied by the weight and divided by 3600, and the square root of this figure is calculated, as illustrated in Figure 6.1.

Stop and Think …

What does the BSA abbreviation stand for?

Describe how you confirm that the dose of chemotherapy you are due to administer.

Area Under the Curve (AUC)

Not all SACT is dosed using BSA. For example, carboplatin dosing is calculated using the AUC, which refers to the target drug exposure over time, instead of dosing based

Body Surface Area Calculation

$$BSA = \sqrt{\frac{H \times W}{3600}}$$

Example: Patient measurements - Height: 1.7m (170cm) / Weight: 65 kilograms

$$\frac{170 \times 65}{3600} = \frac{11050}{3600} = 3.0694 \text{ (rounded 3.07)} \quad \sqrt{3.07} \approx \underline{\mathbf{1.75m^2}}$$

Figure 6.1 Body surface areas calculation

Dose (mg) = Target AUC x (GFR + 25)

Target AUC is determined by the treatment protocol

GFR (Glomerular Filtration Rate) reflects the kidney function

+25 is the non-renal clearance of carboplatin

Figure 6.2 Calvert formula for carboplatin

entirely on body size. This approach is used for carboplatin because the drug is cleared from the body mostly via the kidneys and dosing must therefore take into account the patient's renal function to reduce the risk of toxicity. Carboplatin dosing is calculated using a formula called the Calvert formula (Calvert et al., 1989) (Figure 6.2).

Stop and Think …

What does the AUC abbreviation stand for?

This means that carboplatin dosing is individualised based on kidney function, helping to reduce the risk of toxicity, like bone marrow suppression (BMS), which will be discussed later in this chapter. The SACT competency passport expects all SACT practitioners administering SACT to understand AUC-based dosing, so that calculations can be checked safely before treatment administration.

Dose Banding

Some organisations also use dose banding to reduce calculation errors and improve pharmacy efficiency. Dose banding is used in the delivery of chemotherapy agents such as paclitaxel and docetaxel, as it improves safety by allowing slight variations in BSA-calculated doses to be categorised into agreed dose ranges (a band). For example, if three patients have doses calculated that are very similar, a dose band could be used. An example of how this works is illustrated in Figure 6.3.

There are additional benefits to dose banding, including improved pharmacy efficiency through batch production instead of individualised doses. This reduces drug waste, as multiple bags can be reconstituted from vials at the same time, to reduce the amount of drug thrown away. However, accurate dosing remains vital. If a patient is overdosed, there is an increased risk of both the type and severity of side effects experienced. Equally, underdosing may reduce treatment effectiveness. Dose banding is considered safe for selected SACT treatments, as research has demonstrated that small dose variations of approximately +/−5–10% do not significantly affect treatment effectiveness (Plumridge and Sewell, 2001). Careful consideration is given to dosing in line with governance processes, agreed treatment protocols and the influencing factors outlined in Table 6.2, helping to maintain patient safety and quality of life (QoL).

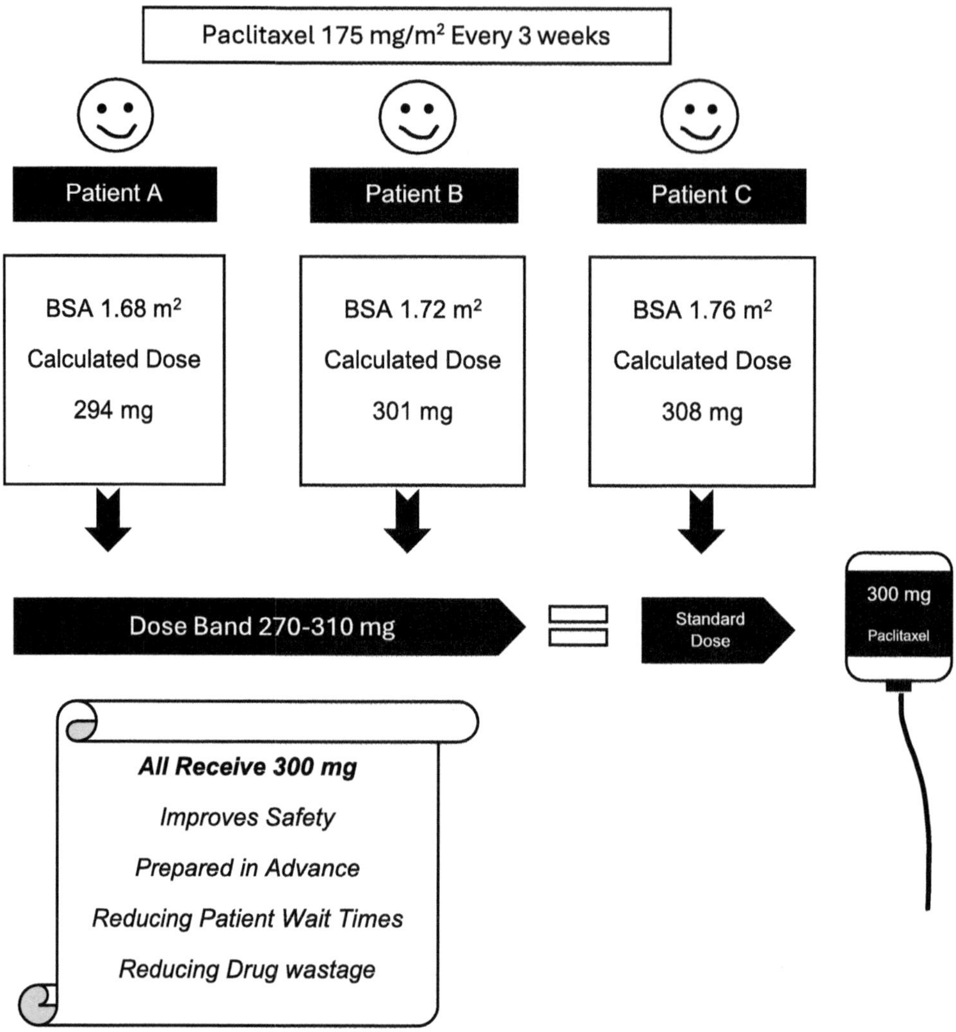

Figure 6.3 Example of dose banding

Vital Signs

Understanding a patient's "norm" helps identify clinical instability and detect early indicators of potential treatment-related side effects. Undertaking a set of observations for all SACT regimens may seem basic, but abnormalities may indicate infection, dehydration and even organ dysfunction, all of which can increase the risk of serious SACT complications. Figure 6.4 outlines some examples that emphasise the importance of identifying issues before treatment, to help ensure the patient is clinically fit to proceed.

Blood Tests

Preparatory blood tests are undertaken to assess the patient's overall health and when considered alongside the patient's performance status (Table 6.2), support the risk assessment process for treatment prescribing and administration. Table 6.3 outlines the

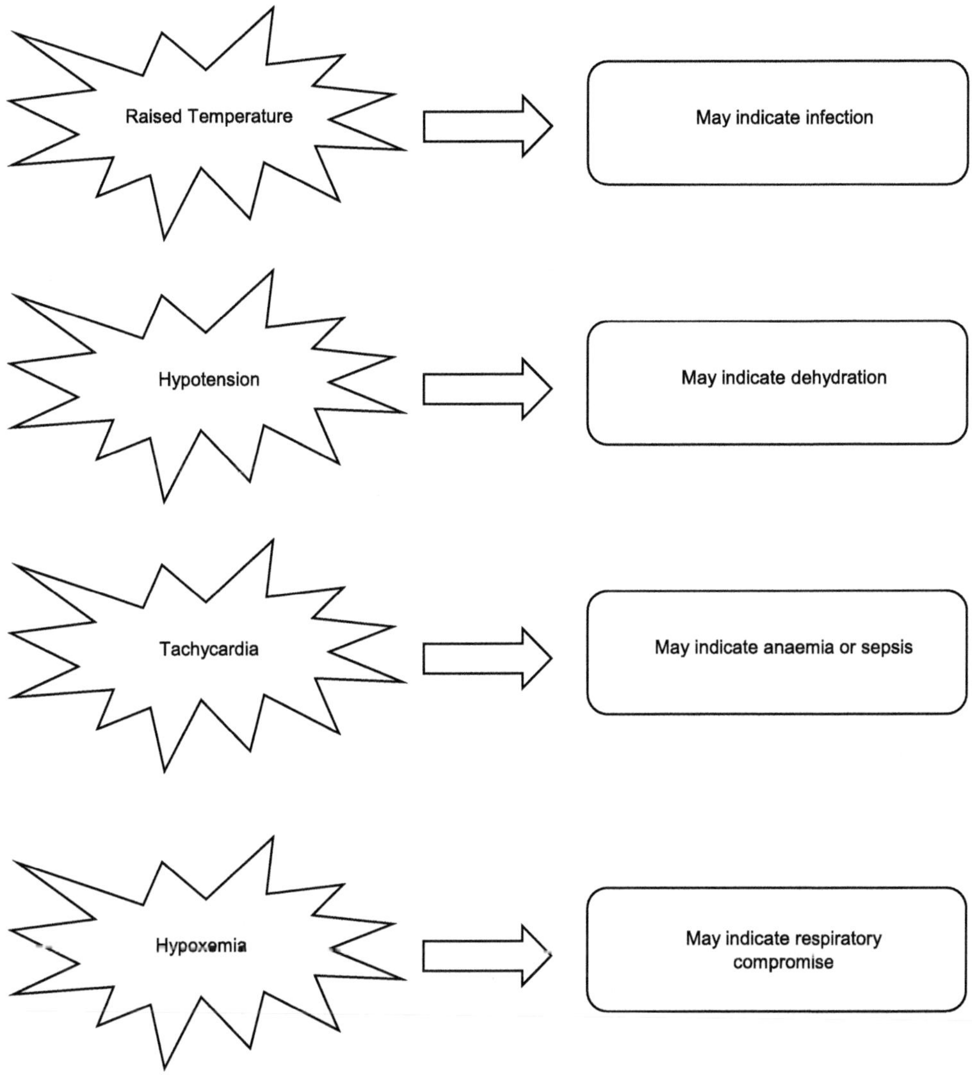

Figure 6.4 Examples of clinical observations and potential indications

initial blood tests required, including normal ranges and the clinical rationale for each. However, it is important to note that the minimum blood levels required to proceed with SACT may vary depending on the treatment protocol.

Lung Function Test

A lung function test may be performed to assess existing lung capacity and identify the risk of pulmonary toxicity. These investigations are regimen-specific and are more commonly required for treatments including:

- Bleomycin
- Methotrexate

Table 6.3 Preparatory blood tests outlining normal ranges and clinical rationale

Blood test	*Normal range*	*Clinical rationale*
Red blood cell	Female: 115–160 grams per litre of blood Male: 130–180 grams per litre of blood	Low Hb may indicate anaemia Increases fatigue risk Reduce tolerance to SACT
White cell count	4–11 × 10^9/L	Leukopenia increases infection risk
Platelets	150–450 × 10^9/L	Thrombocytopenia increases risk of bleeding Treatment delays based on the treatment protocol
Neutrophils	2.0–7.5 × 10^9/L	Most SACT requires ≥1.0–1.5 × 10^9/L to proceed safely
Urea and electrolytes (U&Es) – Renal function test		
Sodium	135–145 mmol/L	Imbalance may worsen with SACT Indicated hydration status
Potassium	3.5–5.0 mmol/L	Abnormal potassium increases risk of arrhythmias with some SACT
Urea	2.5–7.8 mmol/L	Raised urea indicates dehydration or renal impairment
Creatinine	Female: 45–90 µmol/L Male: 60–110 µmol/L	Impaired function increases risk of SACT toxicities when SACT renally excreted
eGFR	>90 ml/min (normal)	Indicates a dose adjustment if <60 ml/min
Liver function test (LFTs)		
Alanine aminotransferase (ALT)	7–56 IU/L	Raised ALT may indicate liver toxicity risk
Aspartate aminotransferase (AST)	10–40 IU/L	Raised AST may indicate liver impairment or metastases
Alkaline phosphatase (ALP)	30–130 IU/L	Raised ALP indicates potential liver metastases or bone disease
Bilirubin	3–17 µmol/L	Assess liver clearance; if raised, it may require dose reduction or treatment delay
Albumin	30–50 g/L	Low albumin is associated with poor treatment tolerance and increased risk of toxicity
Additional tests		
DPYD (genetic test)	Negative/Positive	A positive test would indicate the inability to produce dihydropyrimidine dehydrogenase (DPD) enzyme, which prevents 5-Fluourouracil (5-FU) and Capecitabine from being metabolised, causing a build-up in the body and increased toxicity

Table 6.3 (Continued)

Blood test	*Normal range*	*Clinical rationale*
HbA1C	Non-diabetic <42 mmol/mol Pre-diabetic 42–47 mmol/mol Diabetic: ≥48 mmol/mol	Some SACT treatment increases blood glucose (Steroids, immunotherapy). Poor glycaemic control increases risk of infection and treatment complications
Hepatitis B	Negative/Positive	Some SACT treatments (Rituximab, Steroids, Immunotherapy) can cause Hepatitis B to reactivate, leading to life-threatening complications

- Immunotherapy
- Gemcitabine

Treatment protocols usually outline when a lung function test is required. Reduced lung function at baseline increases the risk of pneumonitis, pulmonary fibrosis and other treatment-related respiratory toxicities. This means when abnormalities are identified, dose reductions or alternative treatments may be considered, if available.

Electrocardiogram (ECG)

Best practice recommends that all patients undergo an ECG before SACT administration, regardless of the regimen. This is to establish if there are any pre-existing cardiac abnormalities, identify arrhythmias or conduction abnormalities and detect baseline QTc prolongation. Without a baseline, it is difficult to determine whether ECG changes during treatment are treatment-related or pre-existing. Performing an ECG prior to treatment supports treatment decisions and safe prescribing, avoiding cardiac complications.

There is a high risk of QTc prolongation with some SACT agents, which increases the risk of life-threatening arrhythmias. Examples of SACT associated with QT prolongation include ribociclib, osimertinib, vandetanib and arsenic trioxide. With ribociclib in particular, the manufacturer guidance is to perform an ECG prior to treatment start, Day 14 of cycle 1 and at the beginning of cycle 2, then additional monitoring if clinically indicated.

Echocardiogram (ECHO)

An ECHO is often performed to assess the baseline cardiac function and measure left ventricular ejection fraction (LVEF) before cardiotoxic SACT. An ECHO is commonly recommended for patients receiving

- Trastuzumab (herceptin)
- Anthracyclines (doxorubicin, epirubicin)
- Pertuzumab
- Some tyrosine kinase inhibitors (TKIs)

An LVEF ≥ 50% is required to proceed with treatment, although this varies with treatment protocol. If cardiac function declines, patients may experience heart failure, cardiomyopathy, fatigue, dyspnoea and fluid overload. Baseline and ongoing cardiac monitoring supports early identification of cardiotoxicity and helps the delivery of safe treatment.

Stop and Think ...

Describe the significance of assessing the physiological function of the organs prior to administering SACT.

Patient Education and Side Effect Management

The importance and mode of delivery of patient education is discussed in Chapter 4. However, in relation to side effects, effective information provision is particularly important. Explaining the common side effects associated with a patient's treatment regimen not only prepares them for what they may experience (returning to the card game analogy) but also allows them to plan and implement self-management strategies. For example, encouraging patients to maintain good hydration, especially in the first few days following treatment, may help reduce the severity of certain side effects such as fatigue, headaches, dizziness and constipation. Dehydration is common during cancer treatment due to nausea, vomiting, diarrhoea and reduced oral intake. This can increase symptom burden and negatively impact the patient's well-being. Maintaining good hydration helps support physiological function and may reduce treatment-related symptom severity (Hwa and Kull, 2020). Providing this information empowers patients to take a proactive role in managing their symptoms and may help reduce avoidable complications, as recommended within the National Cancer Plan for England (Department of Health and Social Care and NHS England, 2026).

In addition to general symptom management strategies, patients must also be informed about treatment-specific side effects, which may impact QoL both during and beyond treatment. For example, some SACT regimens such as taxanes and platinum-based therapies may cause peripheral neuropathy, resulting in numbness, tingling or reduced sensation in the hands and feet. If the neuropathy is severe, it is likely to worsen over the course of treatment. For example, patients can have difficulty fastening buttons when dressing. Early recognition is important, as worsening neuropathy may require dose modification or treatment delay to prevent a decline in QoL. Other treatment-specific regimens can cause alopecia, which can be distressing for both men and women. Preparing patients in advance allows them to explore options such as wig fitting, head coverings or scalp cooling where appropriate.

Reproductive and fertility considerations should be discussed before treatment, especially for patients of childbearing age. Some SACT treatments may affect fertility, either temporarily or permanently. Therefore, discussions regarding sperm banking, egg freezing or embryo storage should take place early on, allowing patients to make informed decisions before treatment starts. In addition, another consideration, which requires discussion not isolated to the younger patient, is the importance of protective sex during and after SACT treatment, for those who still have a libido, to reduce the risk of transferring SACT via bodily fluids, causing injury. However, it should be discussed that patients may also experience a loss of libido. These conversations can be complex and emotionally challenging and, in some cases, embarrassing for the patient, but they are an essential component of holistic patient education and shared decision-making.

In addition to the common side effects, patients must be informed about potentially serious complications, such as neutropenic sepsis or hypersensitivity during administration and extravasation risk. The aim is not only to inform patients of these risks, but also to ensure they understand the associated red flag symptoms. For example, the development of pyrexia may indicate neutropenic sepsis (see Chapter 7), while pain, redness and swelling around the cannula site during intravenous (IV) SACT administration may suggest extravasation (see Chapter 3). Finally, it is essential to ensure each patient receives an alert card and understands its purpose when accessing urgent care. The alert card should include:

- Treatment information
- Emergency contact information (24-hour advise line, inclusive of out-of-hours is different)
- Warning symptoms requiring urgent assessment (Temperature ≥ 37.5, uncontrolled diarrhoea)
- Time critical safety statement (This patient is receiving ... and may develop life-threatening complications ...)

Patients with SACT toxicities can deteriorate very quickly and patients should present this card to staff within emergency departments, GP practices, walk-in-centres and ambulance services, to aid healthcare professionals in these settings, who may not be familiar with SACT treatment and toxicities. They bridge the gap in knowledge to help improve patient safety by prompting urgent medical attention, like antibiotics within one hour (door to needle time) for neutropenic sepsis. By providing this alert card and the education around the importance of seeking medical attention when required, it reassures patients that they are not a burden and are not wasting staff time. It conveys the message that they are able to access help at any time, promptly, should red flag symptoms develop, reducing the risk of death (NCAG, 2009).

Monitoring and Assessment During SACT

General Principles of Toxicity Assessment

Monitoring patients during treatment is essential for tolerability and safety. It is not a one-off event and must occur before each treatment cycle. How this is done differs between organisations. Nevertheless, all areas where SACT is delivered have a systematic approach to this assessment, which often reflects the UKONS triage tool, underpinned by the Common Terminology Criteria for Adverse Events (CTCAE) grading system (Table 7.2, Chapter 7). As a minimum, each assessment should include:

- A review of common treatment-related side effects
- Blood test results
- Performance status assessment

These elements support the overarching clinical question: Is it safe to proceed with treatment today? Potential outcomes to this question are outlined in Figure 6.5.

The SACT practitioner undertaking the assessment must document the findings clearly and accurately, including any actions taken or decisions not to act, with a clear clinical rationale. Accurate documentation supports continuity of care, multidisciplinary communication and patient safety. It also provides an essential record should care delivery be reviewed through a governance process or formal investigation. But importantly, this structured assessment supports a person-centred approach to care planning. By focusing on the patient's current condition, symptoms and treatment tolerance, decisions are

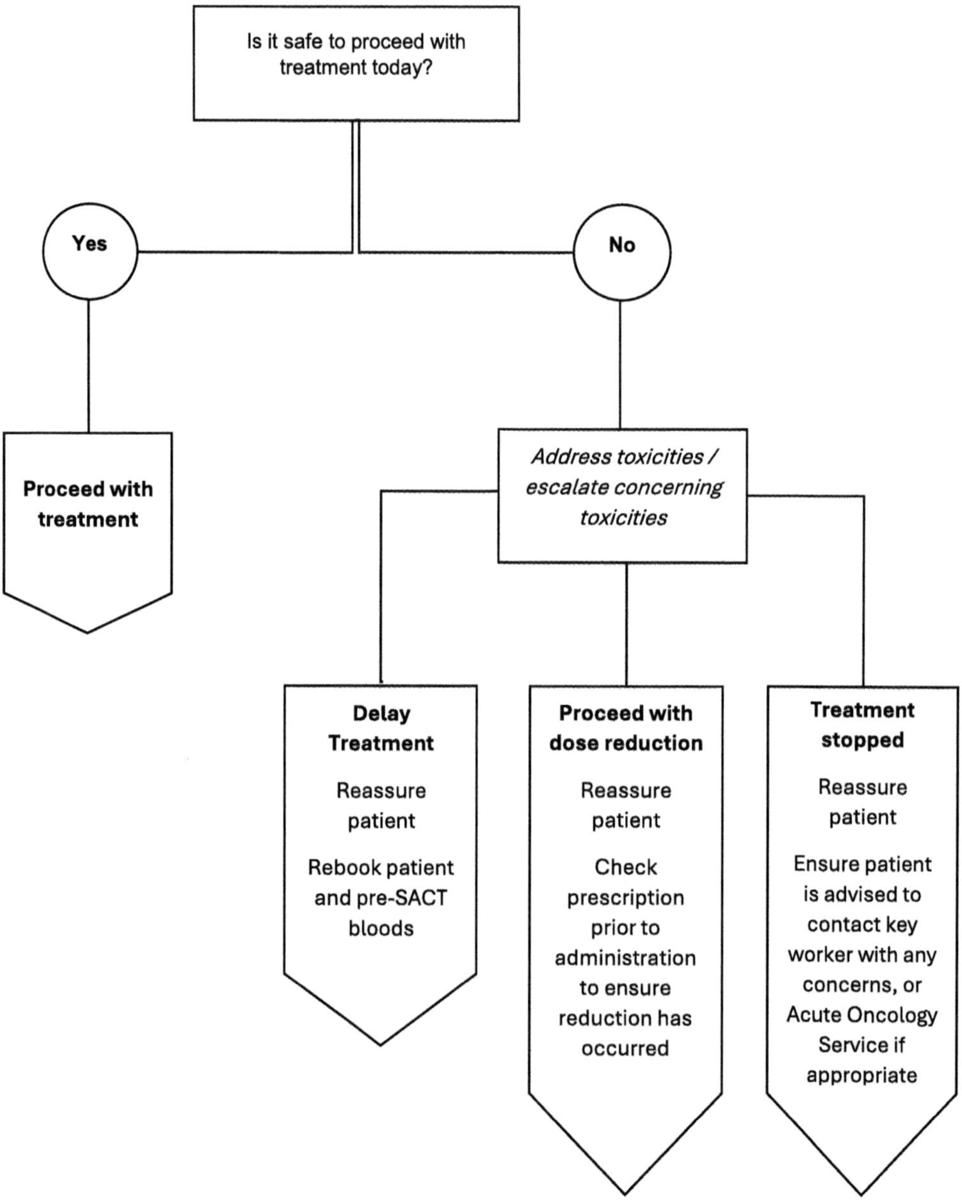

Figure 6.5 "Is it safe to proceed with treatment today?"

made based on individual patient needs, rather than following a purely procedural 'tick box' approach to treatment delivery.

Effective communication during the assessment is also essential. If patients perceive that questions about side effects are being asked solely to determine whether treatment will proceed, they may downplay their symptoms, particularly when they view SACT as their main opportunity for disease control or survival. This can increase the risk of significant toxicity and compromise patient safety. Therefore, SACT practitioners should ensure that patients understand the purpose of the toxicity assessment, that the main aim is to deliver treatment safely and maximise the outcomes. Detecting side effects and managing them early avoids treatment delays, dose reductions, or discontinuation. However, when one of these treatment modifications is necessary, patients should be supported to understand the clinical rationale behind these decisions. These decisions are not taken lightly, with the overall aim to prevent severe or life-threatening toxicity, which in some cases can lead to treatment-related mortality rather than death from the underlying cancer. Clear, compassionate communication is therefore essential to support shared decision-making and maintain patient trust throughout the treatment pathway. This conversation absolutely sits within the remit of the SACT practitioner during treatment assessment and a transparent, open approach should be adopted. This supports shared decision-making, promotes patient understanding and agreement with the treatment plan (concordance) and aligns with professional responsibilities, including the principles of duty of candour.

Common SACT Side Effects: Assessment and Management

BMS

The bone marrow produces blood cells that are essential for immunity, transporting oxygen and clotting. However, when SACT is administered, it targets rapidly dividing cells (as mentioned earlier), including red blood cells (RBC), platelets, white blood cells (WBC) and neutrophils (a type of WBC). This can lead to BMS, also known as myelosuppression, which may result in complications affecting a patient's QoL and in some instances, require additional supportive therapies between treatment cycles, as it can become life-threatening (Figure 6.6). It is important to note that although neutrophils are a subtype to the major blood cell line of WBC, they are also heavily monitored during SACT administration due to their role in infection prevention and the high risk of neutropenic sepsis (see Chapter 7).

In some cases, BMS can affect all three major blood cell types at the same time (RBC, WBC and platelets), this is known as pancytopenia. Pancytopenia is particularly important to watch out for, as patients may experience symptoms of anaemia, increased risk of infection and bleeding, which requires an urgent clinical assessment and treatment plan.

BMS is mostly detected through a blood test, however, there are also other clinical signs and symptoms that healthcare professionals should be aware of, as outlined in Table 6.4. Recognising these early warning signs and symptoms enables the multidisciplinary team to manage these complications quickly to prevent life-threatening deterioration. For example, if neutropenic sepsis is not recognised and acted upon, there is a high risk of organ failure leading to death (see Chapter 7).

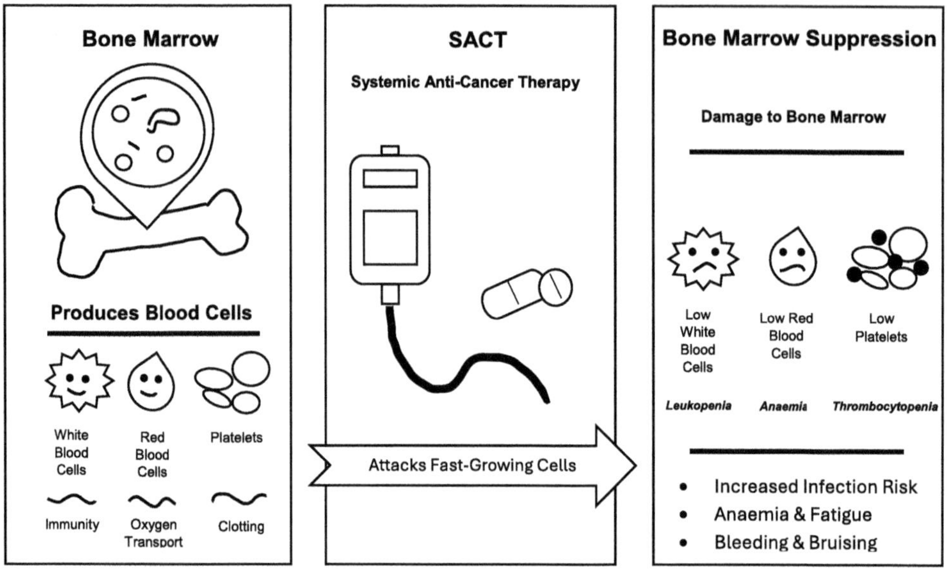

Figure 6.6 Why BMA occurs in SACT

Table 6.4 Signs and symptoms of bone marrow suppression and its potential impact on patients

Blood cell	*Medical term when depleted*	*Signs and symptoms*	*Potential impact*
Red blood cells	Anaemia	Fatigue Shortness of breath Dizziness	Blood transfusions Delayed treatment Reduced quality of life
Platelets	Thrombocytopenia	Bruising Increased risk of bleeding Purpuric rash	Platelet transfusion Delayed treatment Social impact
White blood cells	Leukopenia	Often asymptomatic initially then: Flu-like symptoms General malaise	Treatment delay Increased risk of infection due to overall reduced immune system
Neutrophils (type of WBC)	Neutropenia	Pyrexia Rigors Hypotension Tachycardia	Delayed treatment Intensive care unit admission Death Social impact due to isolation

Table 6.5 Potential holistic management of bone marrow suppression

Condition	*Potential intervention*
Anaemia	• Red blood cell transfusion • Encourage rest • Improving nutrition and hydration • Patient education on when to seek help
Thrombocytopenia	• Advise to avoid activities which could cause injury • Avoid sharp razors (use electric razor) • Avoid NSAIDs (if clinically appropriate) • Monitor for nose bleeds (head forward, pinch bridge of nose, ice pack on forehead, back of neck) • Monitor for unexplained bruising • Patient education on when to seek help • Consider platelet transfusion if appropriate
Leukopenia/Neutropenia	• Growth factors (GCSF – see Chapter 7) • Prophylactic or therapeutic antibiotics (if required) • Antifungal and antiviral therapy for some patients • Patient monitor temperature daily (as per policy) • Good hand hygiene • Avoidance of people with known infection • Food hygiene and safe food preparation • Patient education on when to seek help and neutropenic sepsis (prompt reporting of pyrexia)

Obtaining a blood sample and reviewing the results alongside the toxicity assessment before treatment administration is essential. SACT is generally not reconstituted or ordered, until it is confirmed that the blood results are within the normal range or the acceptable parameters outlined in the treatment regimen protocol. This is not only about reducing potential drug wastage if treatment cannot proceed, but ultimately to ensure patient safety, avoiding further complications or morbidity.

If BMS is identified in a patient prior to treatment, there are several potential management interventions that can be considered, as illustrated in Table 6.5. Before making any formal pharmacology decision, the SACT practitioner must discuss the overall assessment with the prescribing clinician, or most appropriate clinician, to ensure a suitable treatment plan is formulated.

Stop and Think …

Describe the symptoms a patient may experience due to bone-marrow suppression.

Nausea and Vomiting

Nausea and vomiting (N&V) are among the most common and distressing side effects of SACT. These symptoms can significantly disrupt day-to-day life, affecting oral intake, hydration, nutritional status and overall QoL. When N&V is poorly controlled, there is a likelihood of anticipatory nausea, treatment delays, dose reductions, or discontinuation of treatment, potentially impacting treatment outcomes (Hesketh et al., 2020). N&V occur due to the stimulation of multiple pathways within the body, including chemoreceptor trigger zone (CTZ) in the brain, vomiting centre in the medulla oblongata, the gastrointestinal (GI) tract, the vestibular system and higher cortical centres (linked to psychological factors such as anxiety and expectation). SACT agents stimulate the release of neurotransmitters such as, serotonin (5-HT3), dopamine and substance P (NK1 receptor pathway). These neurotransmitters activate the vomiting centre, which instructs the body to physiologically experience N&V (Hesketh et al., 2020).

The severity of N&V is dependent on several factors:

- Type of SACT and its emetogenic potential
- Dose intensity
- Combination SACT regimens
- Patient-related risk factors
- Previous experience with N&V

SACT drugs are classified according to their emetogenic potential, this helps guide prophylactic antiemetic prescribing:

- High emetogenic risk (platinum-based therapy)
- Moderate emetogenic risk
- Low emetogenic risk
- Minimal emetogenic risk

This classification is based on international antiemetic guidelines, such as those developed by MASCC and ESMO, which are used across SACT services to support evidence-based antiemetic prescribing (Herrstedt et al., 2024). Figure 6.7 illustrates how each of these pathways is stimulated and why this occurs, providing an overview of associated signs and symptoms and the types of N&V.

Types of N&V

There are three main types of vomiting associated with SACT, as outlined in Table 6.6. Understanding the type of N&V can help identify the underlying cause and guide appropriate treatment interventions.

Holistic Patient Support

SACT nurses are best placed to assess patients and recognise the impact that N&V can have on their overall well-being. Through therapeutic conversations, practitioners can explore not only the potential causative factors but also provide holistic support and practical advice to help patients manage these distressing symptoms. For example, patients are often advised to avoid eating their favourite foods around the time of treatment. This is important not only because some SACT drugs, particularly platinum-based drugs, can cause taste changes, but also due to the psychological impact of N&V.

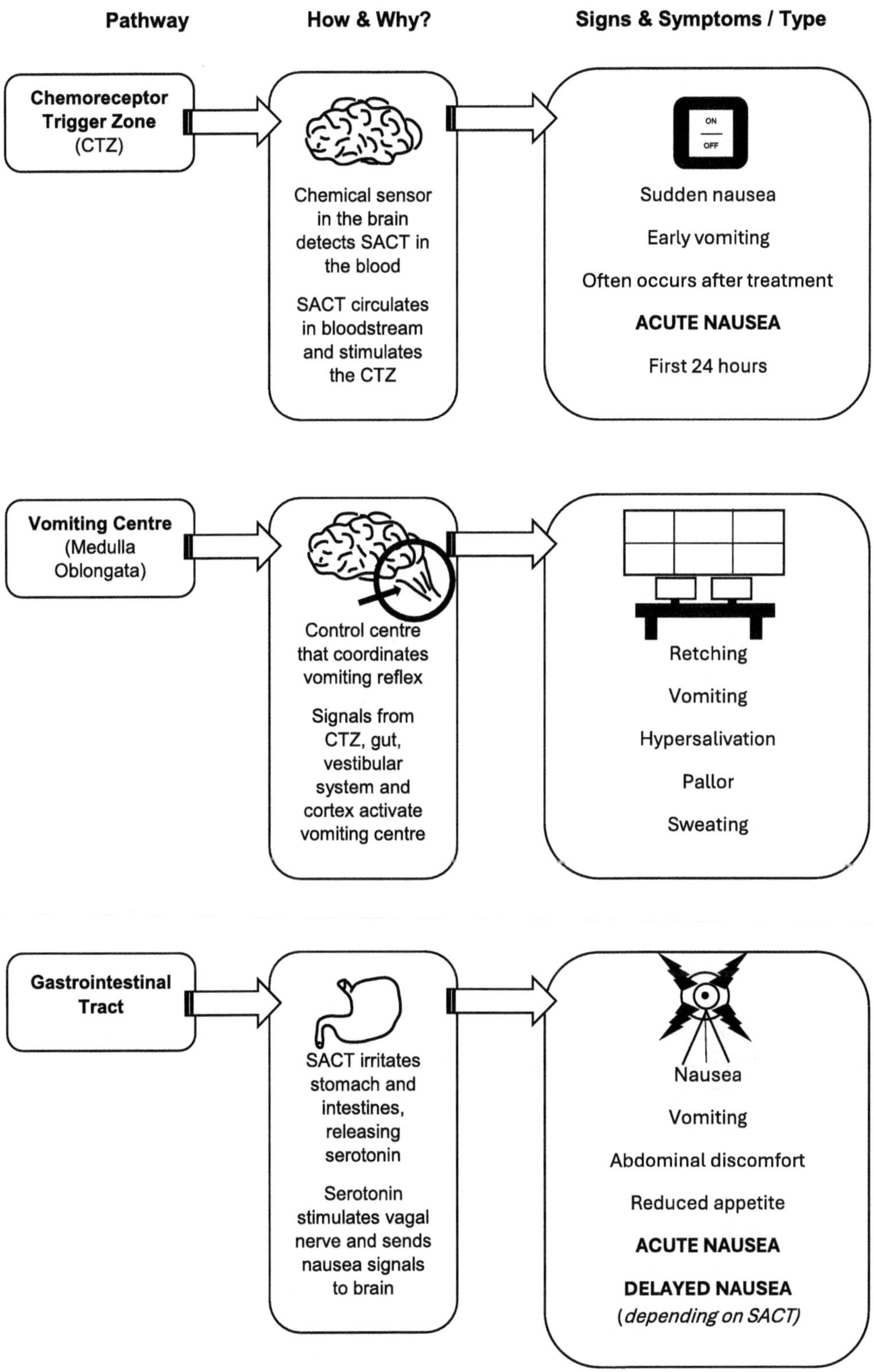

Figure 6.7 How and why pathways are stimulated, highlighting signs and symptoms and type

Table 6.6 Types of N&V, onset, duration and commonalities

Type	*Onset*	*Duration*	*Commonalities*
Acute	Within 24 hours of SACT, commonly within 1–2 hours	Short-lived	Often linked to serotonin release in the gastrointestinal tract
Delayed	Occurs after 24 hours of SACT	May last 2–5 days	Common with Platinums, Cyclophosphamide and Anthracyclines Associated with Substance P (NK1) pathway
Anticipatory	Occurs before treatment Triggered by smells and previous negative experiences	Psychological response, varies with patient	Common if previous nausea poorly controlled Prophylaxis not always effective

If a patient feels unwell after eating their favourite food, they may begin to associate that food with nausea (Cancer Research UK, 2023). Over time, this can lead to food dislikes, where previously enjoyed foods then become unappealing or even trigger feelings of nausea. Providing this simple advice can help preserve appetite and maintain nutritional intake during treatment.

In addition, SACT practitioners should demonstrate empathy and compassion when caring for patients experiencing N&V. Small environmental factors can significantly influence how a patient feels. For example, wearing a strong perfume or aftershave, although pleasant in other settings, may be overwhelming for patients receiving SACT. Consider your practice and the length of time spent in proximity during SACT delivery and how heightened sensitivity to smells can exacerbate nausea. Even everyday factors, such as lingering food odours, including garlic, may magnify their symptoms. Being mindful of these considerations helps create a more comfortable treatment environment and ensures that SACT practitioners do not unintentionally increase a patient's discomfort. Thoughtful, patient-centred care, combined with clinical knowledge, can make a significant difference to the patient experience during SACT treatment.

Assessment of N&V

Effective assessment of N&V is essential to identify complications, such as dehydration, malnutrition and treatment delays. Assessments should include the severity, the frequency, its impact on oral intake and any associated symptoms like abdominal pain. More importantly, SACT practitioners should identify red flag symptoms and ensure patients are aware of when and how to seek medical advice. The CTCAE can support structured assessment. Table 6.7 outlines a holistic approach to assessment.

Table 6.7 Assessment process of N&V

Assessment area	*What to assess*	*Clinical considerations*
Severity	Grade 1–4	Use the patient's description Assess impact on daily activities of living
Frequency and type	Number of vomiting episodes Duration Any patterns	Identify if 'acute', 'delayed' or 'anticipatory' nausea Determine if symptoms are worsening over the treatment duration
Impact on intake	Reduced oral intake Reduced fluid intake Weight loss Signs of dehydration	Assess risk of malnutrition Monitor for dehydration (fluid chart) Consider IV fluids
Associated symptoms	Abdominal pain Constipation Fatigue Headaches	Consider alternative causes
Clinical red flags	Inability to keep fluids down Reduced urine output Dizziness Electrolyte imbalance	May require an urgent review Consider admission or IV management Escalate according to organisational policy
Additional considerations	Previous response to antiemetics Current medications Performance status Anxiety levels Additional causes: infections, brain metastases	Helps guide antiemetic selection Identifies non-SACT causes Supports holistic assessment

Management of N&V

The management of N&V should include prophylactic, rescue and supportive interventions, both pharmacological and non-pharmacological. Organisational policies are best placed to outline this in full, along with treatment protocols as antiemetics are regimen-specific. The following tables will provide a basic outline of the management using prophylactic pharmacological interventions (Table 6.8), rescue antiemetics (Table 6.9) and non-pharmacological interventions (Table 6.10).

Escalation

An in-depth assessment is essential to support the patient. However, recognising when to escalate is equally as important. Escalation may trigger:

- IV antiemetics for severe symptoms
- IV fluids for dehydration

Table 6.8 Prophylactic pharmacological interventions

Antiemetic class	*Examples*	*Mechanism of use*	*When typically used*
5-HT3	Ondansetron Granisetron Palonosetron	Block serotonin release from GI Tract	Acute N&V
NK1 Antagonists	Aprepitant (Emend) Netupitant (Akynzeo)	Block substance P pathway	Delayed N&V High-risk SACT regimens
Corticosteroids	Dexamethasone	Enhances antiemetic effect	Acute and delayed N&V
Dopamine Antagonists (also rescue)	Metoclopramide Prochlorperazine	Dopamine receptor block	Breakthrough nausea
Other options	Olanzapine Cyclizine Haloperidol (specialist use)	Multiple receptor pathways	Complex nausea

Table 6.9 Rescue antiemetic interventions

Situation	*Management approach*	*Example*
Nausea occurs despite prophylaxis	Prescribe rescue antiemetic	Add dopamine antagonist
Breakthrough symptoms	Use of alternative class where possible	If 5-HT3 is used prophylactically, try metoclopramide
Persistent nausea	Escalate to combination therapy	Add additional antiemetic class

- Electrolyte correction
- Treatment delays or dose modifications
- Hospital admission where clinically indicated

Early recognition and proactive management of N&V can significantly improve patient QoL, maintain nutritional status and support the continuation of treatment (see Chapter 7).

Diarrhoea

Diarrhoea is a common side effect of SACT and occurs mainly due to damage caused to the rapidly dividing cells of the GI mucosa. This results in injury to the intestinal lining, reduced absorption of fluids and nutrients, increased fluid secretion into the bowel and inflammation of the GI tract (enteritis), all of which contribute to the development of diarrhoea (Benson et al., 2004). Diarrhoea may also lead to further complications, including dehydration, electrolyte imbalance and an increased risk of infections such as

Table 6.10 Non-pharmacological interventions

Support/advice	*Intervention*	*Clinical rationale*
Hydration advice	Encourage oral fluids Small frequents sips Consider IV fluids if dehydrated	Prevent dehydration Better tolerated during nausea For moderate to severe symptoms
Dietary advice	Small frequent meals Bland foods Cold or room temperature foods Dry foods (dry crackers) Ginger & mint Avoid: • Fatty foods • Spicy foods • Strong smelling foods • Large meals • Rich or heavy foods	Smaller portions easier to tolerate Reduce gastrointestinal irritation Fewer smells for tolerability Better tolerated if nausea is mild Relieve discomfort in the stomach
Environment	Fresh air Sitting upright after meals Avoid lying flat	Reduces nausea triggers Improves gastric emptying Reduces reflux and nausea
Psychological support	Relaxation techniques Distraction Referral to counselling Acupressure bands	Reduces anticipatory nausea Reduces focus on symptoms Psychological symptom control Alternative therapy to relieve N&V

Sources: Ryan et al., 2012; Li et al., 2022.

Clostridioides difficile, especially where antibiotics have also been administered, further disrupting normal flora of the gut.

Diarrhoea is defined as the passing of loose or watery stool more frequently than is usual for the individual, often accompanied by a sudden urgency. Symptoms may occur at any time, including overnight and in severe cases may lead to faecal incontinence. Additional signs and symptoms of SACT-related diarrhoea may include abdominal cramping or discomfort and bloating. Prolonged diarrhoea can also lead to dehydration, which can be indicated with signs of a dry mouth, reduced urine output, dizziness and fatigue. Prompt recognition and management of diarrhoea in patients receiving SACT is essential to prevent further complications, avoid treatment delays and reduce the risk of a hospital admission. This said, there are "red flags" with SACT-induced diarrhoea, which must be addressed urgently. The red flags and their causative factors are noted in Table 6.11

Patients receiving SACT should be advised to contact their 24-hour SACT advice line immediately if any red flag symptoms occur, as early intervention can prevent complications, treatment delays and hospital stays (see Chapter 7). Red flags aside, diarrhoea is assessed before each cycle of SACT, as early identification of severity and potential causes can prevent complications. As previously mentioned, a therapeutic

Table 6.11 Red flag symptoms of diarrhoea in patients receiving SACT

Red flag symptoms	*Why it occurs*
≥4–6 episodes of diarrhoea above baseline in 24 hours	Significant mucosal damage to the GI tract leading to increased secretion and reduced absorption of fluids
Persistent diarrhoea lasting >24 hours	Ongoing GI mucosal inflammation and inability of bowel to recover
Fever (≥38°C)	Possible infection, including neutropenic sepsis or *Clostridioides difficile* infection
Abdominal pain or cramping (moderate to severe)	Inflammation of bowel (enteritis/colitis), possible infection or bowel complications
Blood or mucus in stool	Inflammation of bowel lining or possible colitis, including immune-related colitis with immunotherapy
Signs of dehydration	Fluid loss from frequent loose stools leading to dehydration and electrolyte imbalance
Nocturnal diarrhoea	More severe gastrointestinal irritation and reduced bowel control
Diarrhoea with neutropenia	Increased risk of serious infection due to immunosuppression
Inability to maintain oral intake (either food or fluid)	Severe gastrointestinal irritation leading to nausea, diarrhoea, and dehydration risk

Source: UKONS, 2023.

relationship with the patient is paramount, due to the risk of downplaying symptoms to avoid treatment delays. It can sometimes be of help to advise patients to keep a diary of their bowel habits, as sometimes diarrhoea is cyclical and can be more easily managed if symptoms can be predicted. Recommending the use of the Bristol stool chart can help the patient recognise the different types of stools. When this is coupled with tracking the frequency of bowel movements and shared with the SACT practitioner, it can significantly improve the management of diarrhoea.

The management of diarrhoea in patients receiving SACT focuses on symptom control, prevention of dehydration and maintaining continuity of treatment where appropriate. Table 6.12 identifies both pharmacological and non-pharmacological interventions for SACT-induced diarrhoea in the non-emergency setting.

When considering the management plan for diarrhoea, organisational management guidelines should be followed. To ensure the management of diarrhoea is effective, patients need education on symptom monitoring, staying hydrated and encouraged to report worsening of symptoms, as this prevents the patient from deteriorating and developing further complications. A structured approach supports safe, proactive management of diarrhoea, helping to maintain patient safety, well-being and continuity of treatment.

Constipation

Constipation in patients receiving SACT is commonly associated with certain treatments such as vincristine, paclitaxel and platinum-based therapies, which disrupt normal GI

Table 6.12 Pharmacological and non-pharmacological interventions for SACT-induced diarrhoea

Management approach	*Intervention*	*Clinical rationale*
Pharmacological	Loperamide (1st line)	Reduces bowel motility and controls diarrhoea
	Codeine phosphate (2nd line)	Further reduces bowel motility if symptoms persist
	Octreotide	Gastrointestinal secretions in severe cases
Non-pharmacological	Hydration	
	Encourage increased oral fluid intake	Replaces fluid loss and prevents dehydration
	Fluid balance	Identifies early dehydration
	Dietary	
	Eat small, frequent meals	Reduces burden on the gastrointestinal tract
	Choose bland, low fibre foods	Minimises bowel stimulation and improves tolerance
	Avoid spicy, fatty or high-fibre foods	Prevents further gastrointestinal irritation
	Avoid caffeine and alcohol	Reduces bowel motility and fluid loss

Source: UKONS, 2023.

movement. However, constipation is not only caused by SACT itself, but also due to the use of medications to prevent or manage other treatment-related toxicities, for example:

- Medications (opioids for pain management and some antiemetics, eg. 5HT3 antagonists)
- Reduced mobility (fatigue reduces physical activity and slows GI movement)
- Dietary changes (poor appetite and reduced intake slows GI movement)
- Fluid imbalance (dehydration worsens constipation)

Constipation is often identified during the toxicity assessment prior to SACT administration. The SACT practitioner should check for reduced frequency of bowel movements, fewer than three per week, or fewer than the patient's normal pattern; this should be graded according to CTCAE. In addition, reports of straining and hard stools, or a feeling of incomplete evacuation, abdominal discomfort, bloating, overflow and nausea. During the assessment, SACT practitioners must also be alert for red flag symptoms which might indicate bowel obstruction requiring urgent review:

- Severe abdominal pain or distention
- Vomiting
- Blood in stool
- History of bowel obstruction or recent surgery

The management of constipation is multimodal, combining both pharmacological and non-pharmacological approaches. Intervention should be personalised to the patient's needs, tolerance, comorbidities and SACT treatment plan (Table 6.13).

Table 6.13 Pharmacological and non-pharmacological interventions for constipation

Pharmacological	*Non-pharmacological*
• Review current medications for constipation side effects • Laxatives tailored to patient needs (bulk forming, osmotic, stimulant) • Modify or decrease medications contributing to constipation where clinically appropriate	• Encourage hydration and dietary fibre intake (if tolerated) • Promote regular physical activity and mobility • Provide patient education for self-management

Source: UKONS, 2023.

Each patient's response to interventions may vary and should be bespoke to individual needs. SACT practitioners play a vital role in the early identification and intervention, preventing complications and supporting patient comfort during SACT treatment plans. This may also include abdominal x-rays, suppositories or an enema if appropriate.

Mucositis

Mucositis is a common side effect from SACT and in some cases radiotherapy, which can cause patients significant discomfort and pain. Like with many SACT-related toxicities, mucositis develops because SACT targets the rapidly dividing cells. In this instance, SACT attacks the epithelial cells within the lining of the mouth, throat and GI tract. Damage to these cells results in the breakdown of the mucosal barrier, leading to inflammation and the formation of painful ulcerations. Mucositis can have a substantial impact on a patient's QoL, which affects eating, drinking and medication adherence. If left untreated, or if the symptoms are poorly controlled, mucositis may lead to secondary infections, including fungal, bacterial and viral infections. In severe cases, this can result in treatment delays, dose reductions or discontinuation of SACT, which may impact treatment outcomes. Common SACT agents associated with mucositis include:

- Methotrexate
- 5-Flurouracil (5-FU)
- Doxorubicin
- Capecitabine
- High-dose chemotherapy for bone marrow transplant

However, treatment-related factors are not the only contributors to mucositis severity. Several patient-related risk factors may also increase susceptibility, including poor oral hygiene, pre-existing dental or gum disease, age (very young or older patients), nutritional deficiencies, dehydration, smoking and alcohol use and reduced immune function.

Identification and Assessment

Identification of mucositis relies on both the patient reporting their symptoms and clinical observation. Patients may initially describe subtle symptoms such as "my mouth feels a bit sore", "food tastes different", or "my mouth feels dry". These early signs should prompt further assessment, as early identification allows for timely intervention and prevention of progression of mucositis. When undertaking a clinical observation, a SACT practitioner should be making a visual assessment of the oral cavity using a torch, assessing:

- Lips
- Tongue
- Buccal mucosa
- Gums
- Palate
- Oropharynx (if visible)

The practitioner should be checking for clinical signs and symptoms as outlined in Table 6.14.

Many assessment tools are used across organisations to grade the severity of mucositis. Most organisations use either the WHO Oral Toxicity Scale or the CTCAE tool. These grading systems categorise mucositis into four categories:

- Grade 1: Erythema and mild soreness
- Grade 2: Patchy ulceration, moderate pain
- Grade 3: Painful erythema and difficulty with eating and drinking
- Grade 4: Significant pain, minimal intake and/or reduced urinary output

Mild mucositis is usually considered Grades 1 and 2 and can often be managed with early supportive interventions. However, Grades 3 and 4 mucositis require urgent assessment and management, as explored in the SACT emergencies chapter (Chapter 7). Early recognition and proactive management of mucositis is essential to minimise complications, maintain treatment continuity and support patient comfort throughout SACT treatment.

Preventative and Patient Self-Management

Preventative care is key and patients should be educated regarding self-management strategies before starting SACT (outlined in Table 6.15). This helps the patient have a

Table 6.14 Clinical signs and symptoms of SACT-induced mucositis

Clinical signs	*Symptoms*
• Erythema (red, inflamed mucosa) • White or yellowish ulcers • Pseudomembrane (a coating made of dead epithelial cells, inflammatory cells, fibrin and debris) • Bleeding or fragile tissue in severe cases • Lesions may extend from the oral cavity to the pharynx or oesophagus in severe SACT toxicity • Infection (oral thrush or viral lesions)	• Pain or burning sensation in the mouth or throat • Dysphagia (difficulty swallowing) • Dysgeusia (altered taste) • Xerostomia (dry mouth) • Sensitivity to spicy, acidic or hot foods • Pyrexia (severe cases indicating infection)

Table 6.15 Self-management strategies with clinical rationale

Self-management strategy	*Clinical rationale*
Brush teeth gently using a soft-bristle toothbrush at least twice a day	Gentle brushing removes bacteria and debris but minimises trauma to the inflamed mucosa. Maintaining oral hygiene reduces the risk of infection and supports mucosal healing
Use of non-foaming, mild toothpaste (sodium lauryl sulphate-free)	Mild, non-foaming toothpaste helps maintain oral hygiene while reducing irritation and dryness. Sodium lauryl sulphate can irritate the already inflamed mucosa and worsen discomfort.
Rinse mouth regularly, especially after meals and before bed	Regular mouth rinsing removes food debris, reduces bacterial load and helps maintain moisture in the oral cavity, which promotes healing and reduces infection risk
Keep lips moisturised using a water-based lip balm	Dry and cracked lips can act as an entry point for infections, which can increase discomfort. Maintaining lip moisture helps preserve skin integrity and improve comfort.
Maintain hydration	Staying hydrated helps maintain mucosal moisture, reducing dryness and supports tissue healing. Reduces the risk of further complications such as infection and reduced oral intake

better understanding of the importance of prevention and hopefully reduces the risk of mucositis. However, it is important to recognise that with some treatments, mucositis may still occur despite preventative measures.

Additional Preventative Strategies

Other preventative measures include the use of cryotherapy, which involves the patient sucking ice chips before, during and shortly after SACT administration. This causes local vasoconstriction, reducing blood flow (containing the SACT drug), to the oral mucosa and limiting exposure of mucosal cells. This mirrors the science behind scalp cooling. Cryotherapy is often used with:

- 5-Flurouracil
- Melphalan
- High-dose SACT regimens

Although not widely implemented across organisations, growing evidence suggests cryotherapy may reduce the incidence and severity of mucositis in some SACT regimens.

Management of Grade 1 and 2 Mucositis

Once mucositis is present at Grades 1 and 2, the preventative measures are even more important to continue. However, there are some pharmacological and non-pharmacological interventions to consider, as outlined in Table 6.16.

Table 6.16 Pharmacological and non-pharmacological interventions

Type of intervention	*Intervention*	*Clinical rationale*
Pharmacological	Saline mouthwashes	Helps cleanse oral cavity, maintain moisture and promote healing
	Benzydamine mouthwash (Difflam)	Provides local anti-inflammatory and analgesic effect
	Antifungal treatment (Nystatin, Fluconazole)	Treats fungal infections
	Analgesia (paracetamol or mild opioids)	Controls pain and helps improve oral intake
Non-pharmacological	Soft or modified diet	Minimises trauma to the inflamed mucosa
	Cold food and drinks	Provides soothing effect and reduces discomfort
	Avoid spicy and acidic foods	Prevents worsening of mucosal inflammation
	Dietician referral for reduced oral intake	Supports nutritional intake and prevents weight loss

Source: Colella et al., 2023.

However, if a patient is showing signs of Grade 2 mucositis, both the patient and SACT practitioner should increase monitoring, as mucositis can escalate quickly. Patients should be advised to report worsening pain, reduced oral intake and difficulty swallowing, or any signs of infection, such as pyrexia, immediately. Early escalation and intervention may prevent progression to severe mucositis, which can lead to treatment delays, dose reductions or treatment discontinuation. In some cases, interruption to treatment may compromise disease control and adversely affect patient outcomes, especially where treatment intent is curative or disease control is time sensitive. Additionally, severe mucositis may result in complications, such as infection, malnutrition and dehydration, which can further increase morbidity and in rare, but serious instances contribute to mortality.

Stop and Think …

What are the common side effects of SACT?

Summary

In summary, there are many side effects of SACT, although the type and severity an individual patient will experience varies. Preparatory investigations prior to SACT administration are crucial to record a baseline norm for the patient, but also to ensure the patient is fit enough to receive treatment safely. SACT practitioners need to be familiar with the side effects of treatment, the assessment processes and organisational management guidelines to preserve patient safety and maintain QoL through personalised care.

References

Benson, A.B., Ajani, J.A., Catalano, R.B., Engelking, C., Kornblau, S.M., Martenson, J.A., McCallum, R., Mitchell, E.P., O'Dorisio, T.M., Vokes, E.E. and Wadler, S. (2004) Recommended guidelines for the treatment of cancer treatment-induced diarrhea. *Journal of Clinical Oncology*, 22(14), pp. 2918–2926. https://doi.org/10.1200/JCO.2004.04.132

Calvert, A.H., Newell, D.R., Gumbrell, L.A., O'Reilly, S., Burnell, M., Boxall, F.E., Siddik, Z.H., Judson, I.R., Gore, M.E. and Wiltshaw, E. (1989) Carboplatin dosage: Prospective evaluation of a simple formula based on renal function. *Journal of Clinical Oncology*, 7(11), pp.1748–1756. https://doi.org/10.1200/JCO.1989.7.11.1748

Cancer Research UK (2023) Tips for diet problems. Accessed [online] on 30 March 2026. Available at: www.cancerresearchuk.org/about-cancer/coping/physically/diet-problems/managing/tips-for-diet-problems

Colella, G., Boschetti, C.E., Vitagliano, R., Colella, C., Jiao, L., King-Smith, N., Li, C., Nuoh Lau, Y., Lai, Z., Mohammed, A.I. and Cirillo, N. (2023) Interventions for the prevention of oral mucositis in patients receiving cancer treatment: Evidence from randomised controlled trials. *Journal of Current Oncology,* 30(1), pp. 967–980. https://doi.org/10.3390/curroncol30010074

Department of Health and Social Care and NHS England (2026) *The National Cancer Plan for England: Delivering world class cancer care*. GOV.UK

Herrstedt, J., Clark-Snow, R., Ruhlmann, C.H., Molassiotis, A., Olver, I., Rapoport, B.L., Aapro, M., Dennis, K., Hesketh, P.J., Navari, R.M. et al. (2024) 2023 MASCC and ESMO guideline update for the prevention of chemotherapy- and radiotherapy-induced nausea and vomiting. *ESMO Open*, 9(2), 102195. DOI: 10.1016/j.esmoop.2023.102195

Hesketh, P.J., Kris, M.G., Basch, E., Bohlke, K., Barbour, S.Y., Clark-Snow, R.A., Danso, M.A., Dennis, K., Dupuis, L.L., Dusetzina, S.B., Eng, C., Feyer, P.C., Jordan, K., Noonan, K., Sparacio, D. and Lyman, G.H. (2020) Antiemetics: ASCO guideline update. *Journal of Clinical Oncology*, 38(24), pp. 2782–2797. https://doi.org/10.1200/JCO.20.01296

Hwa, Y.L. and Kull, M.R. (2020) The why and how of maintaining hydration during cancer therapy. *Current Opinion in Supportive and Palliative Care*, 14(4), pp. 324–332. https://doi.org/10.1097/SPC.0000000000000526

Li, K., Cai, Y., Xie, S., Zhou, Y., Dong, J., Zhu, Q., Zhang, J. and Qiu, X. (2022) Evidence summary for nonpharmacological management of chemotherapy-induced nausea and vomiting. *BioMed Research International*, 23, 4741193. https://doi.org/10.1155/2022/4741193

National Chemotherapy Advisory Group (NCAG) (2009) Chemotherapy services in England: Ensuring quality and safety: A report from the National Chemotherapy Advisory Group. London: National Chemotherapy Advisory Group.

Plumridge, R.J. and Sewell, G.J. (2001) Dose-banding of cytotoxic drugs: A new concept in cancer chemotherapy. *Amercian Journal of Health System Pharmacy*, 58(18), pp. 1760–1764.

Ryan, J.L., Heckler, C.E., Roscoe, J.A., Dakhil, S.R., Kirshner, J., Flynn, P.J., Hickok, J.T. and Morrow, G.R. (2012) Ginger (Zingiber officinale) reduces acute chemotherapy-induced nausea: A URCC CCOP study of 576 patients. *Support Care Cancer,* 20(7), 1479–89. https://doi.org/10.1007/s00520-011-1236-3

UK Oncology Nurses Society (UKONS, 2023) Acute Oncology Initial Management Guidelines – Version 4.0. Accessed [online] on 30 March 2026. Available at https://ukons.hosting.sundownsolutions.co.uk/

CHAPTER 7

SACT Emergencies

Samantha Toland

Introduction

In this chapter, you will learn the basis of, and how to manage, urgent/emergency situations that are related to SACT. Some of these can happen during or just after administration, e.g. hypersensitivity/anaphylaxis, cytokine release syndrome (CRS), extravasation (see Chapter 3) and some can happen hours/days/weeks after treatment, e.g. neutropenic sepsis, tumour lysis syndrome (TLS) and severe toxicities (immunotherapy-related toxicities are discussed in Chapter 8).

Acute Oncology Services are often best placed to manage the majority of these following the recommendations within the CAG report (2009), and a set of guidelines has been developed for this (UKONS Acute Oncology Initial Management Guidelines, 2023). However, it is important for all healthcare professionals working with SACT to understand the basis of any emergencies that can occur so that they can manage those that happen during treatment, provide holistic care for patients receiving SACT and provide the appropriate pre-treatment information.

Hypersensitivity and Anaphylaxis

This refers to administration related reactions that tend to occur during or shortly after administration of the drug. They can be immune-mediated (such as in hypersensitivity or anaphylactic reactions) or non-immune mediated (anaphylactoid reactions e.g. cytokine release syndrome which will be explored later in this chapter).

Anaphylaxis

Anaphylaxis is a severe, life-threatening form of hypersensitivity reaction whereby airway and/or breathing and/or circulatory problems arise (Resuscitation Council UK, 2025). It is primarily mediated by immunoglobulin E (IgE) antibodies which are produced following initial exposure to a drug. These antibodies then bind to mast cells

DOI: 10.4324/9781003516477-7

and basophils, sensitising them to future exposure. When these cells are subsequently exposed to the same drug, they degranulate releasing a variety of compounds including histamine, prostaglandins, leukotrienes and cytokines. These compounds are responsible for triggering the symptoms of vasodilation, bronchospasm and increased capillary permeability leading to angioedema and swelling. Typical features include airway/breathing difficulties (e.g. stridor, wheeze, dyspnoea, hypoxia), circulatory signs of shock (pale, clammy, hypotension, tachycardia, dizziness) and skin reactions such as flushing, urticaria (hives) and swelling. Some patients may also have a sense of impending doom as the reaction starts to take hold.

Management of Anaphylaxis

Anaphylaxis should be managed in accordance with the Resuscitation Council UK guidelines (2025). These steps are briefly outlined below:

(A) CALL FOR HELP
(B) Stop infusion
(C) Lie patient flat, with leg elevation if possible (unless patient is struggling to breathe or is pregnant). Patients should not be stood up during or immediately after an anaphylactic reaction due to the risk of postural change (sudden drop in blood pressure).
(D) Administer adrenaline IM as per algorithm. Always inject in the anterolateral aspect – middle third of thigh (through clothing if needed).
(E) Administer oxygen at 15 litres per minute via a non-rebreathing mask.
(F) Following administration of IM adrenaline, transfer to an acute medical ward or observation area for ongoing care. Observation for 6–12 hours is needed. If no response to two doses of IM adrenaline, follow the guidance for management of refractory anaphylaxis.
(G) If a suspected anaphylaxis reaction has occurred, consider taking timed blood samples for mast cell tryptase testing as follows:
   - a sample as soon as possible after the emergency treatment has started
   - a second sample ideally within one or two hours of the onset of symptoms
   - a third sample after 24 hours

(H) Observe and record the pulse rate, blood pressure and skin condition at time of onset, along with any notable impact on airway.
(I) Report unusual anaphylactic reactions and those for black triangle drugs via an incident form and the Yellow Card reporting site.
(J) Document the symptoms and severity of the reactions.

The patients' treating team should be made aware of the reaction and it is generally not recommended to rechallenge with the same agent; consideration should be given to alternative treatments where possible (UK SACT Board, 2025).

Hypersensitivity Reactions

These reactions can be immediate (within 6 hours of drug administration) which are usually IgE-mediated, or non-immediate (from 1 hour after drug administration, to several days after) which are associated with T-cell dependent reactions. Reactions can be graded as in Table 7.1.

Table 7.1 Grading of severity of hypersensitivity/anaphylactic reactions

	Grade 1	*Grade 2*	*Grade 3–4 (anaphylaxis)*
Airway			Angioedema, periorbital/ facial oedema Stridor
Breathing	No bronchospasm	No bronchospasm	Symptomatic bronchospasm with or without urticarial.
	Shortness of breath with moderate exertion	Shortness of breath with minimal exertion	Shortness of breath at rest
			Respiratory distress limiting self-care ADLS. Wheeze <94% SpO_2 (per NEWS 2 SpO_2 Scale 1)
Circulation	Asymptomatic hypotension	Hypotension (non urgent medical intervention indicated) (less than 20 mm Hg drop from baseline)	Symptomatic hypotension (more than 20 mm Hg drop from baseline)
Disability	Mild pain[a] Mild agitation (mood alteration)	Moderate pain[a] Moderate agitation (mood alteration)	Severe pain[a] Severe agitation
Exposure	Mild dizziness (mild unsteadiness or sensation of movement)	Moderate dizziness (mild unsteadiness or sensation of movement)	Severe dizziness (unsteadiness or sensation of movement limiting ADLs/altered consciousness/collapse)
	Fever ≤ 38 Mild chills (shivering/ chattering of teeth)	Fever > 38–39.9 Moderate tremor of the entire body	Fever > 40°C[b] Severe or prolong chills
	Prunitus (mild or localised)	Prunitus (wide spread and intermittent limiting instrumental ADL	Prunitus (widespread constant limiting self-care ADL)
	Transient flushing or rash (covering <10% body surface area (BSA with or without symptoms)	Transient flushing or rash (covering 10–30% body surface area (BSA with or without symptoms)	Severe rash (covering >30% BBSA with moderate or severe symptoms)
	Mild nausea (loss of appetite without alteration in eating habit)	Moderate nausea (oral intake decreased without significant loss) or vomiting	Severe (inadequate oral intake)

a Pain can be anywhere in the body – eg. chest, back, muscles, joints.

b Always consider the risk of sepsis or a blood transfusion reaction and manage in accordance with local protocols/policy.

Then subsequently managed according to the common terminology criteria for adverse events shown in Table 7.2 (CTCAE V6, 2025).

Recognition is key to prevent a reaction from progressing into a life-threatening event (anaphylaxis). A full ABCDE assessment, followed by management with corticosteroids and antihistamines at Grade 2 can be sufficient to avoid worsening to Grades 3–4. It is important to note that the symptoms described above are not always present, for example, some patients may initially present with back pain and some mild flushing but would be classed as having a Grade 2 reaction and would therefore require treatment.

Patients having a Grade 1–2 reaction can safely be rechallenged with the offending drug, provided the reaction has completely resolved. For most SACT, it is recommended that the drug is restarted at half the original rate for 30 minutes then increased back to the original rate for the remainder of the administration. Subsequent cycles can be given at the original rate with premedications added as appropriate (steroids and antihistamines).

Patient anxiety needs to be taken into consideration, as this may lead to symptoms that can mimic a reaction. Panic attacks can occur when patients have had a previous reaction as they can be extremely anxious of having a further, more serious reaction (or if they have witnessed other patients having reactions to the same drugs). This can make a clear differentiation of symptoms difficult as they may experience the 'impending sense of doom' and may also hyperventilate leading to a suspicion of hypersensitivity. However, in the absence of hypotension, pallor, breathing difficulties/wheeze and swelling it is more likely to be anxiety-related rather than a drug reaction.

Laryngeal Spasm

Laryngeal/pharyngeal dysesthesia is a specific reaction to the drug Oxaliplatin. It tends to occur either during or just after infusion of the drug and is exacerbated by cold surroundings/drinks. The patient's larynx/pharynx becomes paralysed giving them a feeling that they are unable to breathe properly which makes them gasp for breath and can cause panic. This can be managed by providing reassurance and support, giving them a warm drink and a warm pack for them to hold against their neck. It usually subsides within a few minutes to an hour.

Figure 7.2 Overview of CRS grading, symptoms and management

Infusion related reaction

Grade 1	Grade 2	Grade 3	Grade 4	Grade 5
Mild transient reaction; infusion interruption not indicated; intervention not indicated	Therapy or infusion interruption indicated but responds promptly to symptomatic treatment (e.g., antihistamines, NSAIDS, narcotics, IV fluids); prophylactic medications indicated for <=24 hrs	Prolonged (e.g., not rapidly responsive to symptomatic medication and/or brief interruption of infusion); recurrence of symptoms following initial improvement; hospitalization indicated for clinical sequelae	Life-threatening consequences; urgent intervention indicated	Death

Definition: A disorder characterized by adverse reaction to the infusion of pharmacological or biological substances.

Navigational Note: If the reaction is an allergic reaction related to an agent, consider reporting as Immune system disorders: Allergic reaction. Do not report both.

Cholinergic Syndrome – Irinotecan

Irinotecan is a drug commonly used in the treatment of gastrointestinal cancers and has the potential to cause an acute cholinergic syndrome (an over stimulation at a neuromuscular junction due to an excess of acetylcholine). This can result in acute diarrhoea, sweating, abdominal pain, watery eyes and increased production of saliva. Atropine is given as a premedication to prevent this reaction from happening, however should cholinergic syndrome still occur a further dose of atropine can be given to ameliorate symptoms.

Neutropenic Sepsis

Many SACT agents have the potential to cause neutropenia – a drop in neutrophils (a type of white blood cell (WBC)). Neutrophils are extremely important in combating infection as they are the most specialised microbicidal phagocyte (phagocyte meaning 'big eater' – they consume and destroy pathogens that are recognised as foreign invaders), released in large numbers during acute infection. They are the most numerous of the WBCs accounting for over half of the total WBC population and are so important as they are the first on the scene to fight infection.

When the neutrophil count is lowered (which is a common side effect of many SACT agents – particularly cytotoxic chemotherapy) to 0.5×10^9/L or below, a patient is considered to be neutropenic and thus have a much greater risk of becoming septic should they contract an infection.

Neutropenic sepsis is a potentially life-threatening complication of anti-cancer treatment and is defined by The National Institute for Health and Care Excellence (NICE, 2020) as: **a neutrophil count of 0.5 × 109/L or lower and either a temperature higher than 38°C or any symptoms and/or signs of sepsis.**

Neutropenia is associated with a profound impairment in inflammatory response leading to lack or minimisation of the usual signs and symptoms of infection, thus making it difficult to identify when a patient may have an infection or may be in early stages of sepsis. This is why it is so important to emphasise that patients should call their emergency helpline/contact the acute oncology service with any symptoms – even if they do not have a temperature (as this is part of the inflammatory response initiated by neutrophils – if there is a lack of neutrophils, a fever/temperature may not be evident).

Signs of Sepsis

Recognition can be difficult in early stages of sepsis, so it is important to carry out thorough assessment and perform observations immediately on presentation. Clinical features of possible sepsis include tachycardia, tachypnoea, hypotension, fever or hypothermia, increased capillary refill time, mottled or ashen skin, cyanosis, newly altered mental state and reduced urinary output. People with sepsis can sometimes present with non-specific, non-localised clinical features, e.g general malaise, agitation, confusion or behavioural change. If the patient appears unwell, or there is concern from a relative or carer that there is a change in appearance or behaviour this should be considered as possible signs of sepsis.

Management of Neutropenic Sepsis

Neutropenic sepsis is classed as a medical emergency. UK Oncology Nurses' Society (UKONS) initial management guidelines (V4, 2023) dictate that if the patient has:

History of temperature at home or
Temperature > 38°C or < 36°C or
Heart Rate > 90 and/or Respiratory Rate > 20 or Generally unwell. Infective symptoms; Shivering/rigors; Diarrhoea

Immediate management is required with intravenous (IV) antibiotics which is also in accordance with the 'Sepsis Six' bundle **within the first hour** of recognition of sepsis (NICE, 2020). Neutropenic sepsis should always be assumed unless proven otherwise; IV access should be obtained; bloods should be taken and antibiotics administered without awaiting results.

Bloods test should include:

- Full blood count (FBC) (will identify if patient is neutropenic – white cell count may be high or low; thrombocytopenia may indicate disseminated intravascular coagulation (DIC), but may also be SACT or cancer-related)
- Urea, creatinine and electrolytes (U and Es) (may indicate dehydration and/or acute kidney injury)
- Liver function tests (LFTs) (increased bilirubin or alanine aminotransferase (ALT) levels may indicate cholestasis or other liver dysfunction and may be SACT-induced)
- C-Reactive Protein (CRP – inflammatory marker indicative of infection)
- Coagulation screen (if abnormal may indicate coagulopathy/DIC)
- Group and save (in case transfusion required)
- Calcium, phosphate, magnesium, urate
- Blood gas along with blood or plasma glucose and lactate (hypoglycaemia may result from depleted glycogen stores; hyperglycaemia may result from the stress response to sepsis; raised lactate is a non-specific indicator of cellular or metabolic stress and is a marker of illness severity, with a higher level predictive of higher mortality rates)
- Peripheral and central line blood cultures (to identify possible causative organisms)

First-line IV antibiotics in neutropenic sepsis are generally broad-spectrum, beta-lactam monotherapy with piperacillin with tazobactam as the initial empiric antibiotic therapy for patients with suspected neutropenic sepsis if there are no patient-specific or local microbiological contraindications. Patients with a penicillin allergy should be given an alternative regimen, which should be identified in local guidelines. Aminoglycoside therapy (e.g. gentamycin) should be avoided in patients who have received platinum-based SACT in the last week, and vancomycin or teicoplanin can be added if a central venous access device is the suspected focus of infection.

Oxygen therapy should be administered to patients with reduced oxygen saturation (below 92%) or with an increase in oxygen requirement over baseline, to maintain oxygen saturation above 94% (unless this is contraindicated).

IV fluid bolus should be administered to restore tissue perfusion and the patient then closely monitored to enable ongoing management and care depending on clinical needs.

A chest X-ray and additional investigations (e.g. wound swabs, CVAD swab, urine culture, sputum culture, etc.) may be required to help identify the source of infection to enable tailoring of antibiotic therapy.

Patients can deteriorate very rapidly requiring more intensive care and may need transfer to a critical care department if they require access and initiation of inotropes (which increase cardiac output by increasing cardiac contractility) or vasopressors (which increase blood pressure by increasing peripheral vascular resistance), to maintain perfusion pressure and prevent multi-organ failure.

Low-Risk Febrile Neutropenia Pathway and MASCC Scoring

Patients can sometimes be discharged with oral antibiotics provided they are assessed as being low risk for complications using the Multinational Association of Supportive Care in Cancer (MASCC) scoring system. This is a validated risk stratification tool that can help to avoid admission reducing pressures on acute oncology services (UKONS, 2023).

Stop and Think ...

If not detected and managed immediately, why could neutropenic sepsis cause death?

Tumour Lysis Syndrome (TLS)

TLS is a potentially life-threatening complication that can occur mainly in patients receiving SACT for haematological malignancies such as leukaemia or lymphoma. It is caused due to large-scale destruction of malignant cells which leads to the release of intracellular contents and electrolytes into the bloodstream that overwhelm the normal physiological mechanisms of clearance leading to renal dysfunction. This can occur spontaneously in malignancies with a high cell replication rate (e.g. Burkitt lymphoma) but more commonly occurs following the administration of SACT (Chan et al., 2025).

Patients should be assessed for their potential risk of developing TLS before commencing treatment, and should then be risk stratified into low, intermediate or high risk according to the following factors:

- Disease histology (faster developing/advanced stage haematological cancers are higher risk)
- Assessment of disease burden (e.g. if there is high white cell count (WCC) at diagnosis (leukaemia's), multiple nodal involvement, large-sized tumours)
- Patient-related factors, e.g. renal dysfunction or renal involvement, frailty, ability to manage prophylactic strategies such as compliance with oral intake of fluids
- Assessment of pre-existing spontaneous laboratory or clinical TLS
- Treatment-specific SACT agents in certain diseases have a higher associated risk of TLS, e.g. venetoclax in chronic lymphocytic leukaemia (CLL), chimeric antigen receptor T(CAR-T)-cell therapy

New and emerging highly effective novel therapies used in these specific settings have increased the risk of TLS and this needs to be recognised and managed effectively to ensure patient safety.

Prophylaxis for TLS

Prophylaxis is the most important strategy in prevention of TLS. Any patients deemed to be at risk of TLS (from low to high risk) should be given some form of prophylaxis. This includes:

- Oral fluids of at least 2–3 litres daily – if a patient cannot comply with this oral intake, then IV fluids should be considered (particularly if high risk for TLS).
- Patient education on risk of TLS, importance of fluids and risk of other nephrotoxic medications.
- Use of prophylactic medications such as allopurinol (low/intermediate risk) or rasburicase (high risk) – these drugs prevent the formation of uric acid/allantoin which can accumulate causing renal damage.
- Monitoring – this will vary depending upon level of risk and prophylactic strategies but can require blood monitoring up to 3–4 times daily according to the clinical situation.
- Disease debulking prior to SACT, e.g. use of steroids in lymphoma to reduce burden of disease before treatment.

Identification and Management of TLS

TLS can be diagnosed as either laboratory TLS or clinical TLS. Laboratory TLS involves having two or more specific abnormalities including hyperuricaemia, hyperkalaemia, hyperphosphataemia and hypocalcaemia, or 25% change from baseline in any of these. Clinical TLS includes all of the previously described laboratory TLS, as well as: creatinine >1.5 × ULN (upper limit of normal) and/or cardiac arrythmia, and/or seizures and/or sudden death.

Clinical symptoms may include nausea, vomiting, diarrhoea, lethargy, myalgia, muscle cramps, paraesthesia, tetany, seizures, cardiac arrhythmias, syncope and even death (Puri et al., 2020).

Patients diagnosed with TLS should receive vigorous hydration (3 litres per day depending on renal function, clinical and fluid status – the aim is to maintain a urine output of 100 $mL/m^2/h$ in adults).

Treatment of electrolyte disturbance should be managed as per local protocols, and kidney replacement therapy considered if patient is refractory to this. Patients should also be given IV rasburicase for up to 7 days (depending on clinical need) and electrolytes measured every 6–12 hours (or more frequently if needed). Regular clinical reassessment of the patient's fluid balance status and urine output is required to guide ongoing management.

Early identification and management of TLS is essential to prevent the need for acute clinical input and kidney replacement therapy.

Stop and Think ...

When caring for a patient with TLS what would your immediate interventions be? And why?

Cytokine Release Syndrome (CRS) and Immune Effector Cell-Associated Neurotoxicity Syndrome (ICANS)

These reactions are specifically in relation to more recently developed therapies known as bispecific antibodies and CAR-T cell therapy (see Chapter 8). While these drugs have shown significant efficacy in the treatment of haematological malignancies (and some solid tumours), their use is associated with potentially life-threatening toxicities that necessitate specialised monitoring and prompt intervention. CRS and ICANS are particularly critical, requiring timely diagnosis, grading and management.

CRS is an intensified immune response that can happen when T-cells and other immune effector cells are activated by the bispecific antibody drug/CAR-T cell therapy. This results in a systemic inflammatory response characterised by fever, hypotension, hypoxia and/or multiple organ toxicity. It usually occurs within hours to days after the first administration. Institutions should have guidelines for the management of CRS where these drugs are administered, and these generally involve grading of the CRS with subsequent management as outlined in Table 7.1.

Bispecific antibody drugs should be permanently discontinued with a Grade 4 reaction, or if a Grade 3 reaction reoccurs following rechallenge.

While this is a serious and potentially life-threatening reaction, most bispecific antibody drugs can be given safely, and most reactions are Grades 1–2 only (Table 7.3).

Immune Effector Cell-Associated Neurotoxicity Syndrome (ICANS)

The precise physiological mechanisms involved in the development of ICANS are yet to be defined, however it is believed to be triggered by the passive diffusion of cytokines, along with the trafficking of T cells and monocyte recruitment, into the central nervous system (CNS) along with macrophage activation. It frequently occurs alongside or following CRS and is characterised by varying degrees of diffuse encephalopathy, which may include focal neurological signs, intracranial hypertension and seizures. Initial symptoms include diminished attention, language disturbances and impaired handwriting. Other manifestations may involve confusion, disorientation, agitation, aphasia, somnolence and tremors. In more severe cases (Grade >2), patients may experience seizures, motor weakness, incontinence, mental obtundation, increased intracranial pressure, papilledema and cerebral oedema. The syndrome can exhibit a biphasic pattern; the first phase often coincides with high fever and other CRS symptoms, while delayed neurotoxicity – such as seizures or confusion – may arise during the third or fourth week post-treatment.

A baseline assessment should be carried out pre-treatment including cognitive function tests and documentation of any pre-existing neurological conditions. Patients should be monitored for signs of ICANS particularly during the initiation/step-up phase of treatment and graded according to the Immune Effector Cell-Associated Encephalopathy (ICE) Score which is a 10-point neurological assessment tool including:

- Orientation to year, month, city, hospital (4 points total)
- Follows commands (1 point)
- Naming three nearby objects (3 points total)

Table 7.3 Overview of CRS grading, symptoms and management

Grade	*Symptoms*	*Management*
Grade 1	Temperature ≥38° without hypotension or hypoxia	Treatment should be interrupted and neutropenic sepsis protocol followed. IV antipyretic and antihistamine should be administered and fluids and oxygen as needed Consideration can be given to treatment with Tocilizumab (monoclonal antibody that prevents inflammation by inhibition of IL-6) for persistent fever or for high-risk patients Dexamethasone can also be given in the ambulatory setting or if the patient has bone pain (tumour flare)
Grade 2	Temperature ≥38°C hypotension responsive to fluids and/or hypoxia requiring <6 L/min oxygen	Treatment should be discontinued and neutropenic sepsis protocol followed. IV antipyretic and antihistamine should be administered IV fluids bolus 500–1000 mL to maintain systolic BP > 90 mm/kg and oxygen as appropriate Administer tocilizumab Consider dexamethasone 10 mg IV 6 hourly if no clinical improvement after 6–8 hours of 1st tocilizumab dose. Continue until symptoms have resolved If hypotension persistent after 2× fluid boluses and tocilizumab, consider low dose vasopressor ITU should be alerted that transfer may be required
Grade 3	Temperature ≥38°C and hypotension requiring vasopressors and/or hypoxia requiring >6 L/min oxygen	Medical Emergency – Transfer to ICU Discontinue current bispecific Manage fever and constitutional symptoms as per Grade 1 and 2 CRS Administer vasopressors and oxygen as required Administer tocilizumab Start dexamethasone 10 mg IV 6 hourly. If no improvement within 6–8 hours, increase to methylprednisolone IV 1 mg/kg BD. Consider taper once symptoms resolved. Consider Anakinra (another immunosuppressant drug) if no clinical improvement after two doses of tocilizumab and regular high-dose corticosteroid
Grade 4	Temperature ≥38°C and hypotension requiring multiple vasopressors and/or hypoxia requiring CPAP/BiPAP/ventilation	Medical emergency – Transfer to ICU Discontinue current bispecific Manage fever and constitutional symptoms as per Grade 1 and 2 CRS Provide positive pressure support (e.g. CPAP) as needed Administer tocilizumab Administer methylprednisolone 1g/day IV for 3 days. Consider Anakinra if no clinical improvement after two doses of tocilizumab and regular high-dose corticosteroid

Source: Local Trust Guideline, 2024.

- Writing a standard sentence (1 point)
- Counting backwards from 100 in tens (1 point)

Management of ICANS

Management of Grade 1 (ICE score 7–9, awakens spontaneously) or Grade 2 (ICE score 3–6, awakens to voice) involves interruption of the bispecific drug, IV hydration, withholding of oral intake (due to aspiration risk), regular neurological observations, and consideration of medications such as anti-seizure drugs, dexamethasone and Tocilizumab/anakinra if ICANS persists or is associated with CRS.

Grade 3 ICANS (ICE score 0–2, awakens only to tactile stimulus, seizures, focal cerebral oedema on imaging) would require transfer to ITU with the same neurological management as for Grades 1 and 2. For steroid treatment, methylprednisolone 1 mg/kg IV every 12 hours should be considered with tapering when symptoms improve.

Grade 4 ICANS (ICE score 0, un-rousable, prolonged (>5 minutes) or frequent seizures, motor weakness, diffuse cerebral oedema on imaging or symptoms of oedema) would require immediate transfer to ITU, same initial maangement as for Grades 1 and 2 along with steroid treatment using methylprednisolone 1000 mg IV OD for 3 days with tapering when symptoms improve, and hyperosmolar therapy with mannitol should also be considered.

Severe Toxicities

Diarrhoea

Diarrhoea is a side effect of many SACT drugs – this is covered in Chapter 6. However, this can become life-threatening if not managed appropriately, or if not acted upon in a timely manner. Patients need to be informed of the importance of contacting the emergency helpline with any symptoms of diarrhoea, but particularly if they are experiencing this at Grade 3–4 or Grade 2 and higher if on immunotherapy treatment, see Table 7.4.

Patients that have received SACT presenting with Grade 3–4 diarrhoea need to be assessed urgently and admitted into hospital for management as IV fluid resuscitation may be required due to the risk of severe dehydration. SACT must be stopped (some patients may be on oral SACT and continue to take them) and the Acute Oncology Team should be involved to ensure appropriate management. This includes:

Table 7.4 Diarrhoea grading

Grade 2	Increase up to 4–6 episodes a day over baseline or moderate increase in ostomy output or nocturnal movement or moderate cramping
Grade 3	Increase up to 7–9 episodes a day or severe increase in ostomy output and/or any of the following: Incontinence Severe cramping Bloody diarrhoea
Grade 4	Increase >10 episodes a day or grossly bloody diarrhoea

Source: UKONS, 2023.

- Urgent assessment – observations and NEWS score
- Bloods to include FBC, U&Es, Mg2+, LFT, CRP, phosphate, blood gases (arterial or venous) for pH/bicarbonate with severe diarrhoea and potential bicarbonate loss
- Stool sample to rule out infective causes of diarrhoea
- Consider abdominal X-ray
- Elimination of other causes (such as infection, graft versus host disease in transplant patients, secondary to neutropenic sepsis)
- IV fluid resuscitation to replace fluid and electrolytes
- Medication review to stop any other medications contributing to dehydration or worsening diarrhoea (such as ACE-inhibitors/diuretics/NSAIDs)
- Keeping the patient nil by mouth if abdominal pain or distension is present or abdominal X-ray is abnormal
- Administration of anti-diarrhoeal medication with caution and only if infective causes have been ruled out (starting with loperamide then adding codeine if ineffective). If Grade 4 – octreotide by subcutaneous injection can be considered and immediate IV broad-spectrum antibiotic given (even if afebrile)

For patients receiving immunotherapy with Grade 2 diarrhoea-urgent management may be required (see Chapter 8).

Nausea/Vomiting

As a side effect, this is described in Chapter 6. However if this becomes a Grade 3–4 toxicity it can become life-threatening and appropriate management is required with admission to hospital and input from the Acute Oncology Team. See Table 7.5.

For Grade 3–4 nausea and/or vomiting SACT should be withheld and urgent assessment and management is required including:

- Urgent assessment – observations and NEWS score.
- Bloods to include FBC, U&Es, CRP, LFT, Mg2+, Ca2+, glucose, CRP, cortisol, blood gases (arterial or venous) for pH/bicarbonate if metabolic alkalosis (abnormally high tissue pH due to metabolic dysfunction) is suspected. Consider blood cultures if infection suspected.
- IV fluids and electrolyte replacement should be given as appropriate.
- Rule out other causes such as disease-related nausea/vomiting for example with brain or liver metastases, electrolyte imbalance and obstruction. Other medications such as opiates. If receiving capecitabine or 5FU, dihydropyrimidine dehydrogenase deficiency (DPD) (a metabolic disorder condition) should be considered.

Table 7.5 Nausea and vomiting grading

Grade 3 and 4 Nausea	Inadequate or no oral caloric and/or fluid intake
Grade 3 Vomiting	6–10 episodes in 24 hours. Acute hospital assessment indicated
Grade 4 Vomiting	Vomiting – >10 episodes in 24 hours. Life threatening consequences

Source: Adapted from UKONS, 2023.

- Antiemetic should be administered as appropriate in line with local policy. (Consider alternative route of administration of antiemetics, e.g. subcutaneous syringe driver.)
- Contact Acute Oncology/Haematology Team who may consider substitution, discontinuation of oral chemotherapy if appropriate.
- Consider viral causes of vomiting – patient should be isolated unless non-infectious cause has been confirmed.

Stop and Think ...
When caring for a patient with severe nausea and vomiting what would you continue to assess and monitor? And why?

Mucositis

As per previous toxicities discussed here, management of mucositis as a side effect of SACT is explored in Chapter 6. If mucositis develops into a severe toxicity at Grade 3–4, this tends to require urgent assessment and management via the Acute Oncology Team and may necessitate admission into hospital. See Table 7.6.

Management at Grade 3–4 includes:

- Check all blood results and act on abnormalities, e.g. neutropenia or pancytopenia.
- Assess for evidence of dehydration, infection and poor oral intake.
- If receiving capecitabine or 5FU consider DPD deficiency.
- Consider IV access and fluid replacement if needed.
- For analgesia, consider dispersible analgesics, e.g. soluble paracetamol/co-codamol – if no improvement, consider use of opiates.
- Consider S/C syringe driver for severe pain.
- Assess for thrush/candidiasis and arrange for an antifungal agent to be prescribed if required.
- Consider referral to the Speech and Language Therapy team to assess swallowing, and dietician for nutritional management and support.
- For symptomatic relief consider use of ice chips, anti-inflammatory mouthwash and mucosal barrier gel (UKONS, 2023).

Stop and Think ...
When caring for a patient with severe mucositis what would your immediate interventions be? And why?

Table 7.6 Mucositis grading

Grade 3	Painful erythema, and difficulty with eating and drinking
Grade 4	Significant pain, minimal intake and/or reduced urinary output

Source: UKONS, 2023.

Summary

In this chapter, we have looked at a variety of emergency situations that can arise due to SACT, both during administration and after treatment. This includes hypersensitivity and anaphylaxis, laryngeal spasm, cholinergic syndrome, neutropenic sepsis, TLS, CRS and ICANS, and severe toxicities of diarrhoea, nausea/vomiting and mucositis. All healthcare professionals involved in SACT should have a clear understanding of how to manage these urgent situations so they can provide patients with appropriate information and are able to act appropriately should any of these situations arise during treatment.

References

Chan, Y.L.T., El-Sharkawi, D., Shah, P., Chanouzas, D., O'Connor, D., Marks, S.D., et al. (2025) British society for haematology updated guidelines for the diagnosis and management of tumour lysis syndrome in adults and children with haematological malignancies: A focus on patient safety. *British Journal of Haematology*, 207(4), 1248–1258. https://doi.org/10.1111/bjh.70092

(July 22, 2025) *Common Terminology Criteria for Adverse Events (CTCAE) v6.0 (MedDRA 28.0)*. Published Cancer Therapy Evaluation Program Division of Cancer Therapy and Diagnosis National Cancer Institute National Institutes of Health U.S. Department of Health and Human Services, USA.

Local trust guideline (2024) *Guideline for the management of cytokine release syndrome (CRS) and immune effector cell associated neurotoxicity syndrome (ICANS) associated with bispecific antibody treatments*, Worcestershire Acute Hospitals Trust, Worcester.

NICE (2020) *Neutropenic sepsis: Prevention and management in people with cancer*. National Institute for Health and Care Excellence, UK. www.nice.org.uk

Puri, I., Sharma, D., Gunturu, K.S. and Ahmed, A.A. (Jun 14, 2020) Diagnosis and management of tumor lysis syndrome. *Journal of Community Hospital Internal Medicine Perspective*, 10(3), pp. 269–272

Resuscitation Council UK (2025) Emergency treatment of anaphylactic reactions: Guidelines for healthcare providers, available at: www.resus.org.uk/library/additional-guidance/guidance-anaphylaxis/emergency-treatment

UK Oncology Nurses Society (UKONS, 2023) Acute Oncology Initial Management Guidelines – Version 4.0 available at UKONS | Acute Oncology Initial Management Guidelines (last accessed 23 March 2026). https://ukons.hosting.sundownsolutions.co.uk/

UK SACT Board (2025) Anaphylaxis and hypersensitivity reactions: guidance for the management of adults receiving intravenous systemic anti-cancer therapy (SACT) for the treatment of solid tumours Version 1.0 8th August 2025, available at: www.uksactboard.org/_files/ugd/638ee8_b05f2c4fff6c4f33b6592a3b53f130e1.pdf

CHAPTER 8

Immunotherapy

Alison Simons

Introduction

This chapter will explore the basics of the immune system and identify the types of immunotherapy drugs that are currently used to treat cancer. How these drugs work on a cellular level will be explained and a rationale for the side effects of those drugs will be included. Assessment of side effects will be explored and the importance of side effect assessment and management discussed.

The Immune System

To be able to understand how these drugs work, we need to understand the basic immune system. The goal of the immune system is to protect the body from pathogens. It consists of innate and adaptive immune systems, the innate being the inbuilt system, for example the skin or gastric acid, and the adaptive system being the more complex part which involves the lymphocytes and has a memory. Overall it's a complex system and relies on different cells, tissues and organs to prevent the entry of pathogens. When pathogens attack, two main types of white blood cells get released: granulocytes, phagocytes (the neutrophils, macrophages and lymphocytes) See Figure 8.1.

Lymphocytes (T cells and B cells) are the focus of immunotherapies. This chapter will explore T cells because these are the cells that are harnessed to attack cancers. T cells are made in the thymus; they can recognise antigens on the surface of pathogen cells, bind to the pathogen and induce apoptosis (cell death). We have discussed in previous chapters that cancer results from DNA mutation and DNA alteration. T cells also play an important part in the recognition of DNA damage or DNA alteration and so can recognise cancerous cells as part of this process. However, some tumour cells express proteins that can block the immune system's ability to recognise them and prevent the T cells from attacking them. Immunotherapy drugs assist the T cells in being able to find and destroy these cancer cells (see Figure 8.2).

DOI: 10.4324/9781003516477-8

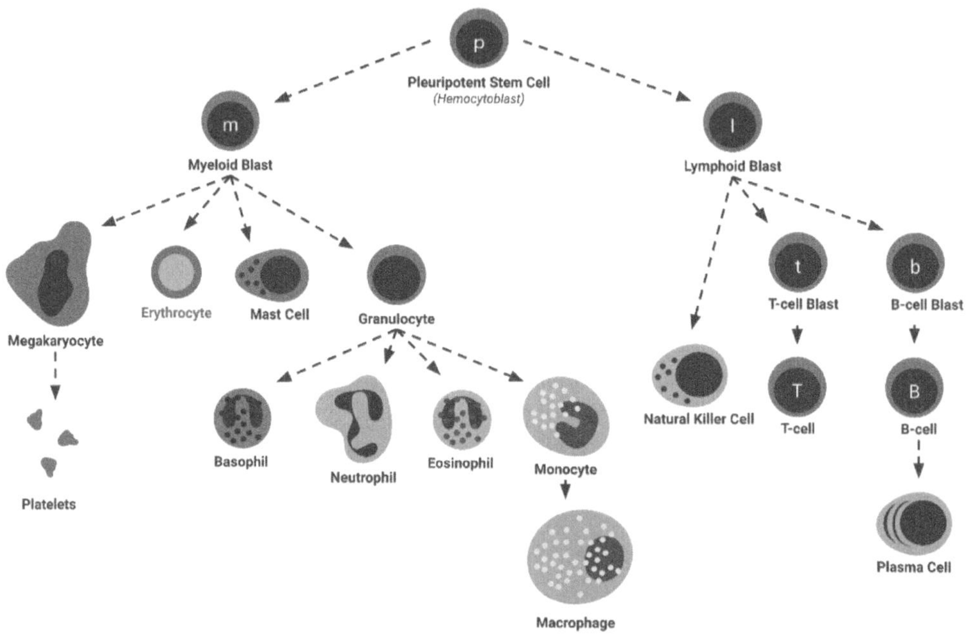

Figure 8.1 The different cells of the immune system

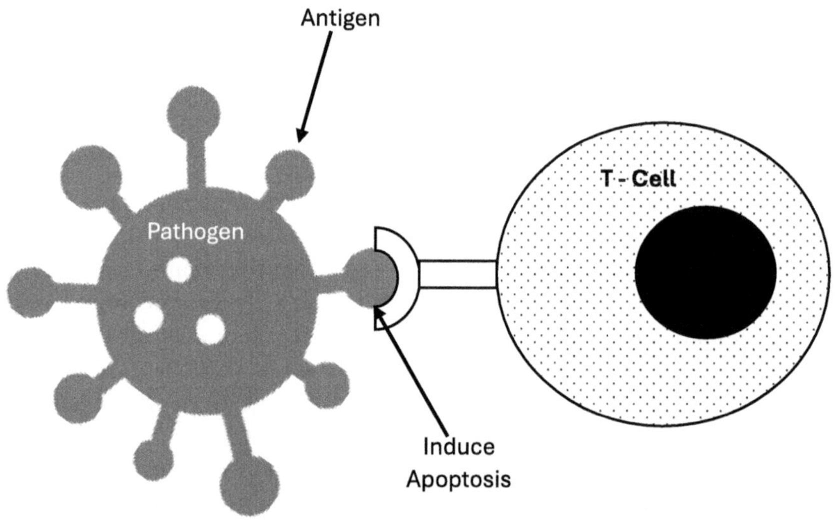

Figure 8.2 A T cell identifying a pathogen and inducing apoptosis

Immunotherapy

Immunotherapy (immuno oncology) refers to the use of medicines or techniques to use the immune system to treat or prevent cancer. Immunotherapy is not a new treatment; it has been around for quite a long time. In the 19th century German and American scientists and medics used streptococcal bacteria to shrink down tumours. Whilst there was some small amount of success, there were problems and side effects such as sepsis and patients quite often died as a result. But this did create the first idea of harnessing and using the immune system to treat cancers. Whilst we discuss immunotherapies that use T cells in this chapter, immunotherapy can refer to some wider drugs that will stimulate the immune system as well.

It is important to note that although these drugs are not currently classified as hazardous drugs (HD) (see Chapter 5), there is no evidence regarding the risk to health (as no studies on this have been undertaken). However, what we do know is their mode of action and toxicity profile and this would suggest that accidental exposure to these could potentially pose concerns. The same safe handling measures used with SACT agents are strongly advised when handling immunotherapy agents to minimise risk of accidental occupational exposure (see Chapter 5).

Immune Checkpoint Inhibitor Drugs (CPI)

Immune checkpoints are molecules that regulate the immune system, sometimes referred to as gatekeepers. While T cells identify and attack pathogens, the immune checkpoint molecules help to protect normal cells from damage. However, when cancer cells block the immune system recognising them (you could imagine this as donning an invisibility cloak) the immune checkpoint molecules will also prevent the cancer cells from being damaged, as the T cell will see them as 'normal' cells. Immune checkpoint inhibitors do just that, they will inhibit the checkpoint protecting the cancer cells from being identified and attacked by the T cells. You could think of this as the invisibility cloak being removed and the cancer cell becoming unmasked and removing the brakes on the immune system. This means the T cells can now identify and attack the tumour cells. CPIs work in two main ways, one which acts on the unmasking of the tumour cell, and the other mainly affects and activates the T cell. Ultimately immunotherapy works by allowing the immune system to attack the cancer cell.

Immune checkpoint inhibitors are now used to treat most tumour sites and have completely revolutionised treatment of melanoma, and lung cancer, leading to these patients living longer. The administration of this treatment has also evolved making administration easier as they are delivered by short IV infusion and more recently are now being administered by subcutaneous injections.

We will now examine the common CPIs used to treat cancer.

Programme Cell Death Protein-1 (PD-1), Programmed Death Ligand 1 (PDL-1) and Programmed Death Ligand 2 (PDL-2) Inhibitors

Programme Cell Death Protein-1 (PD-1) is an immune checkpoint protein found on the surface of the T cells and cancer cells. Programmed Death Ligand 1 (PDL-1) and Programmed Death Ligand 2 (PDL-2) are immune checkpoints on T cells and cancer cells that stop cancer cells being destroyed. When the PD-1 protein binds to PDL-1 or PDL-2 receptors on the surface of normal and cancer cells it prevents the action of the T cell on the cancer cell, so in other words the cancer cell becomes undetected by the immune system (dons an invisibility cloak) See Figure 8.3.

PD-1 checkpoint inhibitor drugs will block the PD-1 from binding to the PDL-1 or PDL-2, while PDL-1 and PDL-2 checkpoint inhibitor drugs block the PDL-1 or PDL-2 from binding to PD-1 receptors on T cells and cancer cells. This means that the T cells

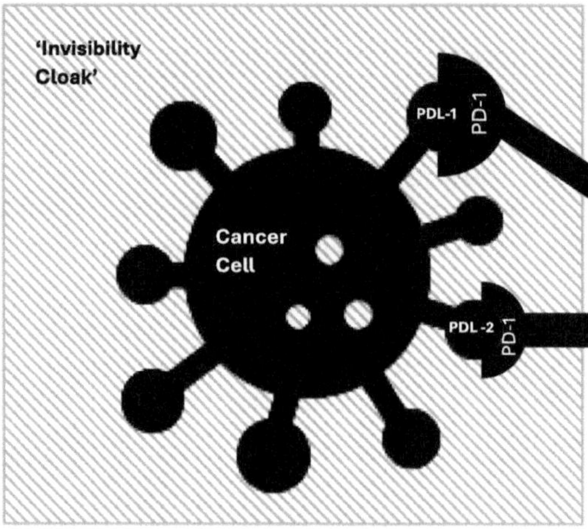

Figure 8.3 PD-1 binding to PDL-1 and PDL-2

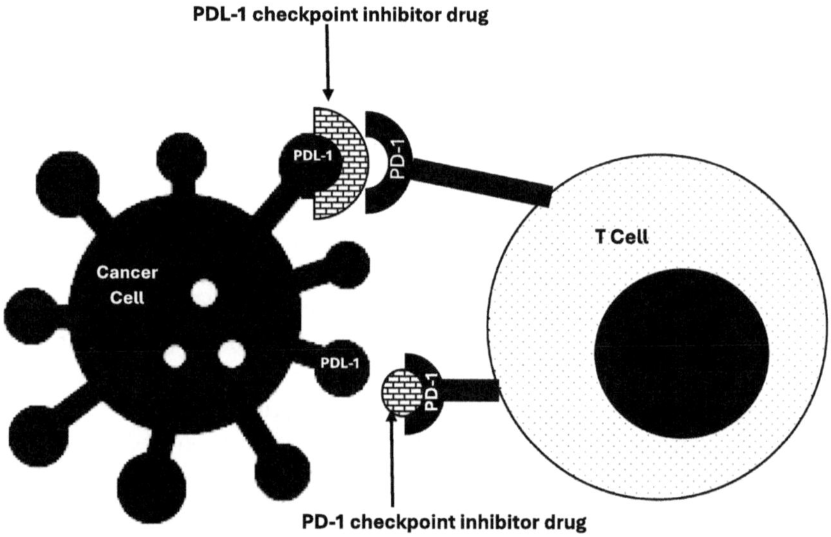

Figure 8.4 PD-1 checkpoint inhibitor drug blocking PD-1 and PDL-1 checkpoint inhibitor drug blocking PDL-1

can now identify and attack those cancer cells. You could think (See Figure 8.4) of these drugs as preventing the cancer cells from donning an invisibility cloak.

Examples of PD-1 inhibitors are nivolumab and pembrolizumab.

Examples of PDL-1 inhibitors are atezolizumab and avelumab.

Cytotoxic T-Lymphocyte-Associated Protein 4 (CTLA- 4) Inhibitors and Lymphocyte Activation Gene 3 (LAG-3) Inhibitor

Cytotoxic T-Lymphocyte-Associated Protein 4 (CTLA- 4) and Lymphocyte Activation Gene 3 (LAG-3) are immune checkpoints that are expressed on specialist T cells, cluster of differentiation 4 (CD4) and cluster of differentiation 8 (CD8). CTLA–4 assists the regulation of the immune response by preventing T cells from killing other cells (including cancer cells). LAG-3 turns off the immune response when required to prevent T cells attacking and destroying healthy cells.

CTLA–4 and LAG-3 inhibitor drugs work by blocking these immune checkpoints and in essence preventing the immune system response being turned off, allowing the T cells to stay switched on resulting in T cells being able to identify and destroy cancer cells.

An example of a CTLA-4 inhibitor is ipilimumab.

An example of a LAG–3 inhibitor is relatlimab.

Stop and Think ...

Describe how you would explain to a new nurse how immunotherapy checkpoint-inhibitors drug work.

Immune-Related Adverse Effects (irEA)

The experience of irEA differs greatly between patients; some patients may experience very mild side effects whilst others may experience multiple severe side effects, as is the case with most anti-cancer treatments. Previously in this chapter we have explored the mode of action of immunotherapy drugs and how they enhance the immune response by turning on the immune system so it can locate and destroy cancer cells that otherwise might have been undetected, however, the difficulty with these drugs is that once the immune response is switched on, it is difficult to switch off that immune response. The immune cells, particularly the T cells, often don't get switched off again and irEA can occur because of this, when T cells become overactive, they start to attack various parts of the body and cause inflammation in any organ or tissues, resulting in a huge number of potential irEA. irEA can present similarly to autoimmune conditions where the immune system destroys its own healthy cells. They can present at varying times, severity and can impact any organ of the body, making predictability and prevention of irEA problematic and in some cases irreversible.

Common IrEA

Cardiovascular

Myocarditis, cardiomyopathy, pericarditis and arrhythmias are some of the cardiovascular side effects from immunotherapy. Cardiovascular irEA have a substantial effect on quality of life and can even be life-threatening.

Dermatological

Skin toxicities are the most common irEA and can range from skin rashes, hair loss and nail changes to more serious conditions such as toxic epidermal necrolysis (TEN). TEN starts with blisters and sores that can occur anywhere in the body including the oral cavity and eyes, and results in large areas of the skin sloughing off. This is due to the immune system cells inadvertently targeting healthy cells within the skin and promoting skin tissue inflammation (Vaez-Gharamaleki, 2025).

Endocrine

The endocrine system is made up of a network of several glands that make and release various hormones. irEA can cause inflammation within any of these glands resulting in dysfunction of the gland that is affected.

Endocrine irEAs include:

- Thyroid-related issues such as either hypothyroidism or hyperthyroidism.
- Adrenal gland-related issues such as adrenal insufficiency, due to the adrenal gland not functioning correctly and not producing sufficient levels of cortisol. Cortisol is a hormone that is often referred to as the stress hormone as it regulates the body's response to stress.
- Pancreatic disorders, particularly diabetes mellitus where the pancreas does not produce sufficient insulin levels. Insulin is a hormone that regulates blood glucose levels.
- Pituitary disorders such as secondary hypophysitis, inflammation of the pituitary gland caused by an external factor, in this case immunotherapy drugs.

Gastrointestinal

Inflammation of the digestive tract (colitis) can occur throughout the whole digestive tract, but particularly in the bowel. Colitis may be so severe that treatment may need to be discontinued. Hepatitis, cholangitis, pancreatitis, oesophagitis and gastritis are other known gastrointestinal irEA.

Musculoskeletal

Rheumatological disorders such as arthralgia, inflammatory arthritis, myalgia and myositis can be due to immunotherapy. This is thought to be due to the functional impairment resulting from inflammatory responses within joints and nerves (Fisher et al., 2025).

Neurological

Inflammation and damage of the nerves block the messages from the nerves to the muscles which causes muscle weakness. This can cause neuropathy, Guillain-Barre syndrome and myasthenia gravis.

Ocular

Ocular inflammation can lead to reduced tear quality causing conjunctivitis and blepharitis, corneal disorders such as dry eye, uvea disorders such as uveitis, retinal disorders such as retinopathies and maculopathies (Wu et al., 2024).

Renal

Checkpoint inhibitor-associated acute kidney injury (IC-AKI) is a lesser common irEA, presenting as a variety of forms of nephritis and cystitis in the main.

Respiratory

Pneumonitis, inflammation and irritation of the lungs is a rare, but potentially fatal irEA. Lung toxicity tends to occur during the first few months of treatment and tends to be more common in patients receiving PD-1/PD-L1 inhibitors (Spagnolo et al., 2022).

Stop and Think ...

Describe how you would explain to a new nurse why irEA may occur and give five examples of the most common irEA.

Management of irEA

Prevention

Previously in this chapter we identified that irEA occur in any type of tissues and organs, are non-site specific, vary in onset timeframes and severity; this makes prevention challenging. Therefore, education of both healthcare practitioners and patients is key.

It would be unreasonable for practitioners to know every irEA, and as the use of this therapy evolves more irEA will be discovered. However, similarly with any medication, awareness of the spectrum of toxicity of the drugs being used is safe practice (Champiat et al., 2016). Having a general knowledge and understanding of the mode of action of immunotherapy agents, particularly in terms of their action on the immune system means that practitioners can identify potential irEA early. Recognising the risk that the immune response may be overactivated resulting in inflammation of healthy tissues is paramount. Being aware of the signs and symptoms of inflammation and being vigilant of these within patients will not prevent them developing irEA but aims to facilitate early identification and management.

Educating patients of the risk of developing irEA is best practice. General information regarding the common irEA, signs to look out for, when and how to get support is key information for patients. This key information also needs to be communicated to the patients' healthcare providers (such as their GP).

Assessment

Reducing the risk of irEA is about being able to recognise if any of those effects are starting to occur, it is important that patients are assessed rigorously before their treatment. The use of an assessment tool is vital, and the UKONS triage tool is recommended in guiding the assessment process. The triage tool lists each toxicity/symptom and offers prompt questions for the assessor to ask the patient, and depending on the patient's response a grade for that toxicity can be identified. The UKONS triage tool uses a numerical and Red Amber Green rating. If amber is indicated in 1 toxicity this would indicate a review within 24 hours, if 2 or more ambers are indicated then this should be escalated to a red rating indicating a face-to-face assessment as soon as possible. This tool was originally developed for assessment of SACT toxicity; it now incorporates other treatment side effects including immunotherapies. The Common Terminology Criteria for Adverse Events (CTCAE) is another tool, which is a set of standardised criteria for defining adverse events using a severity scale range of 1–5. Local guidance should be available on what immunotherapy-specific investigations must be undertaken. Pre-assessment for each subsequent cycle of treatment must include assessment of the risks of the different types of toxicities, for example:

- Dermatological toxicity: assessing for itching, rashes or any skin changes that might indicate dermatitis as a result of the immunotherapy.
- Endocrine toxicity: a range of endocrine bloods, particularly thyroid, cortisol and LH, FSH and testosterone would be expected. However, assessment can be difficult because the symptoms of endocrine toxicities tend to be very vague and wide-ranging. It can be things like fatigue, irritability, headaches, dizziness, changes in mood, behavioural changes, hair loss, feeling cold, constipation, weight gain, weight loss, rapid heartbeat, abdominal pain or hypotension. Including assessment of these symptoms is vital in trying to establish if there is any endocrine toxicity.
- Gastrointestinal toxicity: assessing if diarrhoea has been experienced but importantly what type of diarrhoea this was: has it increased in frequency? Was there any abdominal pain, blood or mucus in the stools, severe abdominal pain accompanying the diarrhoea, or a fever, as these may indicate colitis. It is important that we can pick up the grade of toxicity because that will determine the management.
- Hepatic toxicity: screening for abnormal liver function tests is vital as this may indicate hepatitis. Visual assessment such as any yellowing of the skin or eyes, dark urine, bruising and bleeding may also help to identify hepatic toxicity.
- Musculoskeletal toxicity: Assessment of any severe muscle or joint pains or joint swellings that might be a result of rheumatological inflammation must be considered.
- Neurological toxicity: assessing for any neurological changes, any weaknesses, any sensory alterations or numbness anywhere, may be a result of the immunotherapy.
- Ocular toxicity may cause changes in vision, sore, itchy, dry or weeping eyes that indicate inflammation. Visual assessment of the eye should therefore be undertaken.
- Renal toxicity: nephritis needs to be considered. Assessing for any increase in creatinine, decrease in urine output, haematuria, swelling, is required.
- Respiratory toxicity: assessing if a patient has a cough and or shortness of breath that is getting worse, or experiencing any worsening chest pain is key. However, this can be challenging as many patients receive immunotherapy to treat lung cancer, so may already present with a cough as part of their disease. Utilising any information from standard regular CT scans could help in identifying pneumonitis as a result of the immunotherapy.

Management

Management of irEA should be guided by local policies, procedures and assessment. The specific management will be guided by the severity of the irEA indicated by the grade or score identified in the assessment process. UKONS Acute Oncology Initial Management Guidelines (2023) are designed to offer guidance on the initial assessment and immediate management of Acute Oncology patients (for the first 24 hours). This tool also uses a RAG rating in line with the UKONS triage tool. The management guidelines include detailed individual protocols for the initial management of specific irEAs, identifying the clinical assessments, investigations and treatment required dependent on the grade of severity. Table 8.1 shows a very basic general principle of management of irEAs

Table 8.1 Basic general principle of management

Mild (Grade 1)	*Moderate (Grade 2)*	*Severe or life-threatening (Grade 3 + 4)*
Continue with immunotherapy	Oral steroids Delay immunotherapy	IV steroids Delay or withdraw immunotherapy

dependent on the grade. For more comprehensive and toxicity-specific management, local and national policies and guidelines should be followed.

There are situations which would warrant permanent discontinuation of therapy, for example Grade 3–4 colitis, neuronitis, renal toxicity or skin toxicity. In these situations, patients can become very upset and may still be very keen to stay on the therapy; it is important for them to understand the long and short term risks of continuing with treatment, and that even though they may have only had one or two doses of immunotherapy that it still may be successful and may still have an impact on their disease. Patients can still experience irEAs, 12 to 18 months after they have finished treatment, and up to 2 years in some cases. Whilst on one hand this can be difficult to tolerate and manage, the reassuring thing is that those therapies are still potentially working during that time.

Assessment and management of irEAs are key; if a toxicity can be identified early, for example at grade two, it might mean by withholding therapy we may then be able to continue with it once that toxicity is resolved, so by capturing them early is much more beneficial for the patient. The important thing to remember is that if a patient is receiving immunotherapy and appears with vague symptoms, think autoimmune and get advice, it can be difficult to pinpoint irEAs because they are different to chemotherapy toxicity in terms of severity, drugs and side effects. As a SACT nurse it's vital you are able identify those differences and whether they need any form of treatment.

Other Types of Immunotherapy Treatments

Cytokine Therapy

Cytokines are proteins made in white blood cells, which are involved with cell-to-cell communication during an immune response. Laboratory-engineered cytokines can be given to enhance this mechanism allowing the immune system to identify cancer cells more easily and then destroy them. For example, manmade interferon can activate natural killer cells, which produce enzymes that can help destroy tumour cells. Interferon can also activate dendritic cells which are phagocytes, antigen-presenting cells that act as messengers between the innate to the adaptive immune systems (see immune system section). An example of a man-made interferon is peginterferon. Man-made interleukin boosts the numbers of white blood cells which will increase the immune response against cancer.

Adoptive Cell Transfer (or CAR-T Cell Therapy)

We previously discussed in this chapter that T cells are one of a number of white blood cells that play a part in the immune response to infection and disease. T cells have a

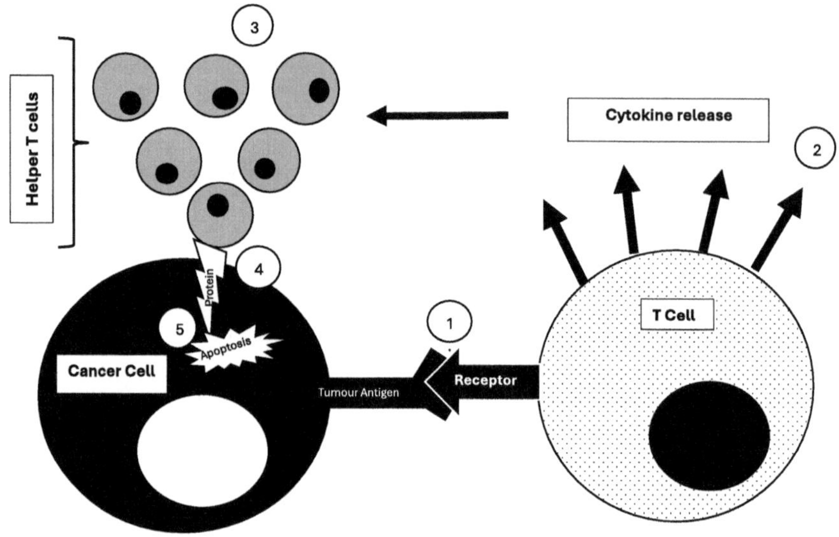

Figure 8.5 Normal T cell activation

Table 8.2 General side effects of CAR-T therapy

- Allergic reaction
- Cytokine release syndrome
- Neurological side effects
- increased risk of infection
- Tumour lysis syndrome

receptor on their cell surface which enables them to lock on to the tumour antigen (markers found on the surface of the cancer cell) and alert the body that a cell is abnormal and action is needed to destroy it. It does this by releasing cytokines which cause other helper T cells to come to the site. These cells then attach to the cancer cell and diffuse it with a protein, which induces apoptosis (cell death) See Figure 8.5.

CAR-T therapy treatment uses a patient's own T cells to enhance the body's response to seek and destroy cancer cells. The patient's T cells are extracted through an apheresis process, (separation of blood components using centrifugal force) and are then genetically modified in a laboratory where chimeric antigen receptor proteins are added to their T cell. This reprograms the T cells to identify and target the cancerous cells more effectively, by enhancing the function of the T-Cell immune response, inducing apoptosis of the abnormal cells (Thoms and Simons, 2024). General side effects of CART-T therapy are shown in Table 8.2.

Bispecific Antibody Treatments

Bispecific antibodies are a more recently developed form of immunotherapy treatment, mainly used in the treatment of haematological malignancies, although they are also being studied in other cancers. T cell engaging bispecific antibodies are designed to simultaneously bind to two antigens for example, T cells via CD3 and surface antigens on cancer cells. This dual binding mechanism activates and redirects T cells against the cancer cell, leading to the release of granzymes, perforins and pro-inflammatory cytokines, which facilitate T cell-mediated cancer cell killing. A variety of bispecific antibodies are currently approved, targeting different antigens on cancer cells. Bispecific agents have demonstrated significant efficacy in the treatment of haematological malignancies; however, their use is associated with potentially life-threatening toxicities that necessitate specialised monitoring and prompt intervention. Similarly to CAR-T cell therapy, among these toxicities are cytokine release syndrome (CRS) and immune effector cell-associated neurotoxicity syndrome (ICANS) which are particularly critical, requiring timely diagnosis, grading and management.

Cancer Vaccines

Vaccines

Vaccines are made from inactive/weak forms of a disease or virus. When a vaccine is administered the immune system is stimulated to develop antibodies to attack this inactive/weak form of the disease or virus. Vaccines harness the adaptive immune system, and as we have previously mentioned in this chapter, it is the adaptive immune system that has memory. This means that if you were to encounter this disease again, the adaptive immune system's B cells would remember the disease or virus and use the antibodies it had developed to be able to attack it, offering protection from developing the disease or virus.

Vaccines to Prevent Cancer

Some cancers have a link to viruses that increase the risk of developing specific cancers, for example the human papilloma virus (HPV) is linked to cervical, vaginal, vulval, anal and penile cancers. This usually means that the virus damages the DNA which can lead to initiation of cancer as described in Chapter 1. Types of head and neck cancers such as mouth or oropharyngeal cancer can also be linked to HPV. Therefore, being vaccinated against HPV significantly reduces the risk of developing HPV, and as a result this will also reduce the risk of developing cancers linked to HPV.

In the case of other cancers, vaccines are used to treat cancer rather than prevent cancer (however this may change in the future due to ongoing research).

Vaccines to Treat Cancer

Bacillus Calmette-Guerin (BCG)

BCG is a vaccine for tuberculosis (TB) that contains a weakened strain of *Mycobacterium bovis* bacteria. BCG has been used to treat contained bladder cancer for three decades; however, the mechanism of action is still unclear. It is thought to be twofold, firstly it can act directly on the bladder cancer cells to induce apoptosis, and secondly it can boost the immune system by the release of killer cells to increase the chances of identifying cancer cells within the bladder and destroying them.

Talimogene Laherparepvec (T-VEC)

T-VEC is a form of immunotherapy that uses a genetically altered weakened form of the herpes simplex virus; this is the virus that is responsible for cold sores.

Summary

In previous chapters we have identified the types of cancers that are treated using specific drugs. Theoretically immunotherapies do not target a specific type of cancer, as these drugs do not target anything within the cancer unlike with traditional cytotoxic chemotherapy. Immunotherapies can therefore potentially impact any type of cancer if the tumour cells express the identified checkpoints included within this chapter (and are licensed for use). It is good news that there is a new set of revolutionary drugs that allow the body to attack the cancer cells itself, that we now have in our armoury to use.

As research advances it is very likely that more checkpoints will be discovered and drugs developed to inhibit these checkpoints.

It is critical that patients are educated and understand the seriousness of toxicities, and the importance of reporting their symptoms promptly. Practitioners need to be able to recognise the early signs of toxicities and be able to manage them quickly.

References

Champiat, S. et al. (2016) Management of immune checkpoint blockade dysimmune toxicities: A collaborative position paper. *Annals of Oncology*, [Online] 27(4), pp. 59–574.

Fisher, B.A. et al. (2025) Immune checkpoint inhibitor-induced inflammatory arthritis. *Clinical Medicine*, [Online] 25(5), pp. 1–4.

Spagnolo, P. et al. (2022) Pulmonary adverse events following immune checkpoint inhibitors. *Current Opinion in Pulmonary Medicine*, [Online] 28(5), pp. 391–398.

Thoms, E. and Simons, A. (2024) Chimeric antigen receptor (CAR) T-cell therapy: An overview for nurses. *Nursing Standard*, [Online] 39(11), pp. 49–54.

United Kingdom Oncology Nursing Society (2023) Acute Oncology Initial Management Guidelines Available Online https://www.ukacuteoncology.co.uk/application/files/9116/9082/2886/UKONS_AO_initial_management_Guidelines_FINAL_VERSION_2023.pdf

Vaez-Gharamaleki, Y. et al. (2025) Dermatologic toxicities related to cancer immunotherapy. *Toxicology Reports*, [Online] 14, pp. 1–28.

Wu, K Y. et al. (2024) Emerging ocular side effects of immune checkpoint inhibitors: A comprehensive review. *Biomedicines*, [Online] 12(11), p. 2547.

CHAPTER 9

Related Therapies

Alison Simons

Introduction

Other therapies used alongside SACT either as treatment for disease or as supportive therapy during SACT will be explained in this chapter. It will include the basic mechanisms of action of these therapies, and some of their side effects. The related therapies that will be explored are targeted therapies, hormone therapy and supportive therapies. Examples of drugs used in the treatment of cancer for each category will be included, however this is not exhaustive, and new drugs are being discovered and implemented all the time, so more recent therapies post-publication will not be included in the examples. A separate chapter is dedicated to immunotherapy drugs.

Targeted Therapies

Targeted therapies are drugs that target a specific protein, process or pathway involved in cancer (Vickers, 2025, pg 62). There are many types of targeted therapy, and they all work slightly differently. In general, some targeted therapies work on the outside of the cell, and others work within the cell. In this section we will look at monoclonal antibodies, growth inhibitors and small molecule inhibitors used to treat cancer, however there is no agreed classification of targeted therapies so this may be categorised in another ways in other literature.

Monoclonal Antibodies (mAbs)

Cancer cells have overexpressed proteins on the surface of their cell. Each specific cancer type has specific abnormal proteins on its cell surface. mAbs work by recognising these specific abnormal proteins. Each mAb can recognise one specific protein and that's why they are often referred to as targeted therapy (See Figure 9.1) as it is targeted at the specific protein on the cancer cell surface.

DOI: 10.4324/9781003516477-9

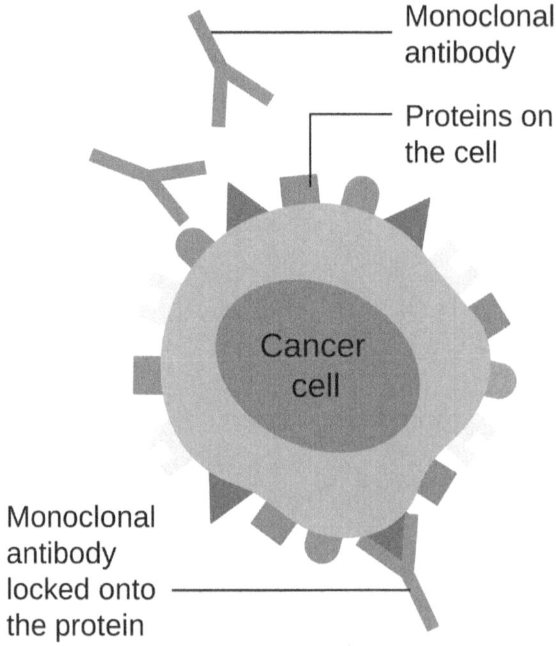

Figure 9.1 Cancer cell with abnormal protein on its surface

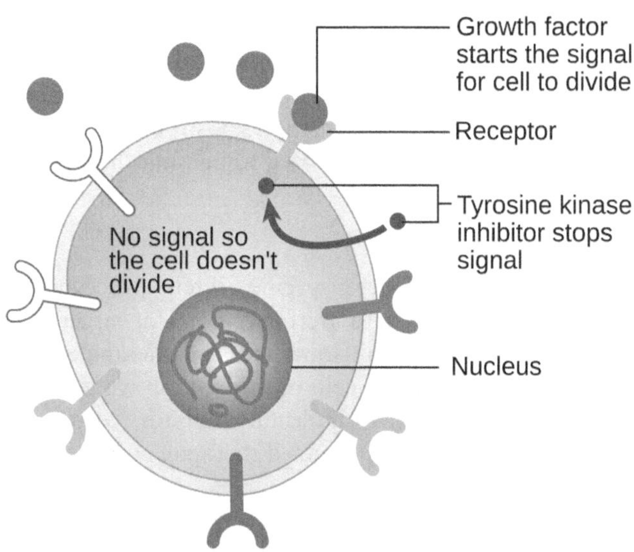

Figure 9.2 Cancer cell with abnormal protein on its surface and the mAbs attaching to it

Once the mAb has identified the specific abnormal protein on the cancer cells surface it will attach itself to it. This works on a lock-and-key hypothesis in that it will only fit that protein; other mAbs will not recognise or be able to attach to that specific protein (see Figure 9.2).

Ultimately, mAbs work by triggering the immune system to attack and kill the cancer cells, (Simons and Cutler, 2013, pg 281) and they work in three slightly different ways. Some mAbs will attach themselves to the proteins on cancer cells to make it easier for the immune system cells to locate them; these are often referred to as flag wavers, indicating where there is a cancer cell that needs attention. Rituximab is an example of a mAb that works in this way.

In Chapter 1 we looked at the control of cell growth and the role of growth factors in this carefully regulated process. Remember we explored that for normal cells to grow and divide, specific growth factors will bind to specific growth factor receptors on the surface of the cells which sets off a signal that tells the nucleus of the cells to divide for that cell lineage. In Chapter 1 we discussed how cancer cells can grow quite rapidly, and they proliferate quickly, this can be due to the cancer cells having many more growth factor receptors on their surface than non-cancerous cells. Having more growth factor receptors increases their chances for increased numbers of growth factors to attach to these receptors and stimulate cell growth. Some mAbs identify cancer cells by looking for cells that have too many growth receptors on their surface. What these mAbs do is attach to these growth factor receptors to block the growth factor being able to attach to the receptor, meaning the cancer cell cannot receive the signal to grow. Pertuzumab is an example of a mAb that works in this way.

Antibody–drug conjugates (ADC) are mAbs that are manufactured to be attached to chemotherapy drugs or radioactive substance particles. This means that when this mAb attaches to the abnormal protein on the cancer cell surface, it will deliver the chemotherapy or radioactive substance particle directly to the cancer cell. ADC can target and deliver treatment to specific cancer cells, and normal cells will not receive treatment, meaning there will be fewer side effects from this treatment. Trastuzumab emtansine is an example of a conjugated mAb that works in this way.

Side Effects of mAbs

Specific mAbs can have infusion reactions and specific side effects (Table 9.1). These infusion reactions and general side effects are typical of immune responses and are due to the way drugs work, in terms of stimulating the immune system to recognise cancer cells. Sometimes there is overstimulation of the immune system and that's when patients may experience these kinds of reactions and side effects. However, symptoms of these reactions and side effects may not always be a bad thing, obviously they can be unpleasant for the patient, but by experiencing some element of these reactions and side

Table 9.1 Common mAb infusion reactions and side effects

Common mAb side effects	*Common mAb infusion reactions*
• Diarrhoea • Fatigue • Nausea	• Flu like symptoms – chills, fever, dizziness • Itchy rash • Breathlessness • Headaches • Flushes and faints Changes in blood pressure

effects does show that the mAbs are actually doing what they're supposed to be doing in terms of their action on the immune system.

Stop and Think ...
Describe how you would explain to a new nurse how monoclonal antibodies work.

Anti-Cancer Small Molecule Inhibitors

Anti-cancer small molecule inhibitors are a group of targeted therapies that inhibit targeted molecules, usually proteins or enzymes, known to contribute to the process of cancer.

Growth Factor Inhibitors

As previously mentioned, growth factors bind to growth factor receptors on the cell surface, which sets off internal signalling to the cell nucleus to instruct it to divide. Tyrosine kinases are enzymes that participate in this chemical message within the cell to the nucleus. Each growth factor is designed to target a specific family of cells, so will only be able to bind to that specific growth factor receptor (See Table 9.2). It's important to note that this is a complex process and no growth factor works alone.

Growth inhibitors aim to slow down or stop this targeted cell growth, and they can work either externally or internally depending on which point of the cell growth process they target. As previously mentioned in this chapter some mAbs can block the growth receptors on the cell surface which inhibit cell growth and can therefore also be classified as growth factor inhibitors.

Tyrosine kinases inhibitors (TKIs) on the other hand work internally within the cell by blocking the action of tyrosine kinase. Tyrosine kinase forms part of the chemical message to the nucleus to instruct cell division, therefore if this message is blocked by the TKI the message to induce cell division cannot be delivered, and therefore cell division does not occur. Imatinib is an example of a TKI.

Table 9.2 Well-known growth factors

Growth factor	*Target*
Epidermal growth factor (EGF)	Growth of epidermal and epithelial cells such as platelet fibroblasts, macrophages
Vascular endothelial growth factors (VEGFs)	Growth of vascular endothelial cells and macrophages
Platelet-derived growth factor (PDGF)	Growth of vascular smooth muscle cells
Colony-stimulating factors (CSFs)	Growth of monocytes, neutrophils, eosinophils, basophils
Erythropoietin (EPO)	Stimulate development of bone marrow erythrocytes

Table 9.3 General side effects of growth inhibitors

- Fatigue
- Diarrhoea
- Skin changes
- Mucositis
- Loss of appetite
- BMD
- Oedema

Growth Inhibitor Side Effects

Each individual growth inhibitor has its own side effect profile. Table 9.3 shows the most common general side effects for growth inhibitors, and these are similar to the general side effects of traditional cytotoxic agents.

Stop and Think …

Describe how you would explain to a new nurse how growth inhibitors work.

Angiogenesis Inhibitors

Angiogenesis is the normal process of the growth of new blood vessels. When a cell does not have a blood supply, it also means they do not receive oxygen, nutrients or growth factors which they need to survive and grow. Without an oxygen supply the cell becomes hypoxic, and this triggers the production of vascular endothelial growth factors (VEGF). In Table 9.2 we identified that VEGF target the growth of vascular endothelial cells and macrophages. In this case it signals the endothelial cells in the capillaries or blood vessel walls to grow and divide. The new epithelial cell growth creates new blood vessels, enabling the hypoxic cell to have a blood supply, providing oxygen, nutrients and growth factors which facilitate cell growth. You could think of this as the hypoxic cell making a telephone call to a taxi or food delivery company to deliver what they need.

The angiogenic process is also active in cancer cells, meaning they can develop a blood supply that not only provides them with the requirements they need to stimulate them to grow, but also provides a mechanism to allow them to spread and infiltrate into the blood system. Once cancer cells can access the blood system, they can travel to other parts of the body where they can metastasise. Using the taxi analogy again this is like calling the taxi to pick the cancer cell up and drive them to another part of the body.

Anti-angiogenic (angiogenic inhibitors) agents block the VEGF signals reaching the epithelial cells within the blood vessels and capillary beds. This means that the message to stimulate epithelial cell growth is not received and cell growth and division does not occur. This results in the cancer cell being unable to receive oxygen, nutrient and growth factors which it requires for cell division and means that they are unable to access the blood supply preventing motility and metastasis. Continuing with the analogy you could think of this as there being no mobile phone signal to make the call to the food delivery service to bring what the cancer cell requires and means they cannot call the taxi to take them to other parts of the body. Bevacizumab is an example of an anti-angiogenic agent.

Stop and Think ...

Describe how you would explain to a new nurse how anti-angiogenics work.

Proteasome Inhibitors

Proteasomes are protease complexes that break down proteins that are no longer required into smaller parts and either reuse them, recycle them for bigger proteins that are required or destroy them.

Therefore, proteasomes regulate the number of proteins within a cell and take action to ensure there are not too many proteins within the cell. Proteasome inhibitors prevent the breakdown of large proteins that the body doesn't require. This leads to a build-up of large proteins within the cell, which causes the cell to become toxic and triggers apoptosis. Bortezomib is an example of a proteasome inhibitor.

mTOR Inhibitors

Mechanistic target of rapamycin (mTOR) is a protein kinase which promotes cell growth. In tumour cells, mTOR is often abnormally activated resulting in cancer cell growth, metastasis and invasion. mTOR is also thought to be heavily involved in the process of angiogenesis, which is the formation of new blood vessels, which in turn provides a blood supply for the tumour and cancer cells which aids cell growth and motility.

mTOR inhibitors stops the mTOR protein kinase promoting cell growth in cancer cells and therefore tumour growth can be inhibited. Everolimus is an example of a proteasome inhibitor.

Phosphoinositide 3-Kinase Inhibitors

Phosphoinositide 3-kinases (Pi3K) are closely related to kinase proteins and are part of a signalling pathway that plays a role in cell survival, proliferation and differentiation. In some cancer cells, Pi3K is permanently switched on, and this causes uncontrolled cell growth, and development of its own blood supply. Once a tumour has its own blood supply cancer cells can metastasise more effectively by using blood vessels as a mode of transport to other parts of the body. Pi3K inhibitors can constrain this, and therefore stop cell growth, cell proliferation, formation of blood supply and motility within cancer cells. Alpelisib is an example of a Pi3K inhibitor.

Histone Deacetylase Inhibitors

In previous chapters we have established that DNA is a tightly wound double helix structure. DNA is wrapped around protein structures called histones which provide the structural support for chromosomes. Histone deacetylases (HDA) are enzymes that aid histones to wind around DNA more tightly providing robust structural integrity for chromosomes.

HDAs also play a role in regulating DNA transcription. It does this by removing the acetyl group from particular proteins which increases the affinity for binding of DNA. This tight packaging of the DNA can limit the transcription of DNA and transcription of genes such as those involved in cell growth and division.

HDA inhibitors (HDI) prevent the action of HDA which leads to relaxation of the DNA helix, allowing transcription of genes that help control cell growth and division. Remember we discussed in Chapter 1 how these genes have a role in instructing apoptosis in cancer cells, so HDA inhibitors can facilitate cancer cell death. Panobinostat is an example of an HDI.

Hedgehog Signalling Pathway Blockers

The Hedgehog signalling pathway is a group of proteins that send signals within the developing embryo. These signals help instruct cells to grow in the right place and in the right way, for example the growth of blood vessels and nerves which is vital within a developing embryo.

Predominantly in adults, the Hedgehog signalling pathway is not active, as this instruction is not needed when we are fully formed. However, in some people, changes in genes can switch on the Hedgehog signalling pathway again, resulting in unregulated cell growth and proliferation increasing the risk of developing cancer.

Hedgehog signalling pathway blockers target the Hedgehog signalling pathway proteins to switch them off and stop the instruction of cell growth. In doing this, proliferation of cells and unregulated cell growth can be minimised. The Hedgehog signalling pathway blockers can also be used to treat cancer. Vismodegib is an example of a Hedgehog pathway blocker.

PARP Inhibitors

Poly ADP-ribose polymerase (PARP) is an enzyme that engages in repairing damaged DNA. They are activated when DNA damage occurs and recruits other repair proteins to promote repair of DNA (Rose et al 2020). PARP inhibitors work by interrupting the PARP enzyme from undertaking cell and DNA repair in cancer cells. As we discussed in Chapter 1, when a cell can't be repaired, apoptosis is induced, leading to cell death. Olaparib is an example of a PARP inhibitor. The general side effects of anticancer small molecule inhibitors are listed in Table 9.4.

Table 9.4 Side effects of anti-cancer small molecule inhibitors

- *Fatigue*
- *Diarrhoea*
- *Skin changes*
- *Mucositis*
- *Loss of appetite*
- *Oedema*

Table 9.5 Common side effects of HITs

- Nausea
- Constipation
- Fatigue
- BMD
- Dizziness
- Mood changes
- Confusion

Histology-Dependent Therapies (HITs)

Most targeted therapies are used to treat a specific type of cancer; however, HITs (or tumour/tissue-agnostic therapy) can be used to treat any type of solid cancer that have a neurotrophic tyrosine receptor kinase (NTRK) gene fusion. The NTKR gene codes for transmembrane proteins; if this gene becomes damaged the proteins they code for can become fused causing unregulated cell growth. HITs work by inhibiting the tyrosine receptor kinase (TRK) which decreases cell proliferation. Larotrectinib is an example of a HIT.

Side Effects of HITs

The long-term side effects of HITs are not yet known; the common side effects are listed in Table 9.5.

Hormone Therapy

Some tumours are sensitive to hormones. Breast cancer can be oestrogen receptor-positive (ER+), meaning they need oestrogen to grow, they can be progesterone-positive (PR+) needing progesterone to grow, or they can be both oestrogen- and progesterone-positive, needing both oestrogen and progesterone to grow. Prostate cancer is testosterone-sensitive, while endometrial cancers are sensitive to oestrogen. Therefore, in terms of hormone therapy for cancer, the aim is to either prevent hormone synthesis or prevent hormones reaching cancer cells.

Anti-Oestrogens (Oestrogen Antagonists or Oestrogen Blockers)

Oestrogen has many functions, but it is responsible for stimulating growth and differentiation of cells within the sexual organs. Breast cancers that are ER+ have breast cancer cells that have oestrogen receptors (ER); these act by binding to oestrogen causing proliferation of breast cancer cells. Anti-oestrogens work by blocking the ER which inhibits or supresses oestrogen production and therefore prevents or reduces the proliferation of breast cancer cells. Tamoxifen is an example of an anti-oestrogen.

Aromatase Inhibitors

Aromatase is an enzyme that turns androgens (precursors of oestrogen) into oestrogen. Aromatase inhibitors block the action of the aromatase enzyme, which means that oestrogen synthesis is halted. This drug is used to treat breast cancer that is ER+ in post-menopausal women; this is when oestrogen is no longer produced by the ovaries and is instead made in the fatty tissue. In premenopausal women, oestrogen is produced in the ovaries at a level that is too high for aromatase inhibitors to work effectively. By preventing the synthesis of oestrogen, this can stop or slow down the growth rate of the ER+ breast cancer cells. Anastrozole is an example of an aromatase inhibitor.

Gonadotrophin-Releasing Hormone (GnRH) Blocker

GnRH (previously known as luteinising hormone-releasing hormone (LHRH)) is a hormone that is released by the hypothalamus (Casati et al., 2023). GnRH stimulates the pituitary gland to secrete the luteinising hormone (LH). LH sends messages to the testicles to make testosterone in males and to the ovaries to make oestrogen and progesterone in females (Casati et al., 2023).

GnRH blockers prevent the hypothalamus making GnRH and thus prevents the pituitary gland making LH and ultimately prevent the testicles from producing testosterone in males and the ovaries to make oestrogen and progesterone in females. GnRH blockers are used in the treatment of prostate in men and breast cancer in women. Degarelix is an example of a GnRH blocker.

Anti-Androgens

Androgens are a group of hormones that include testosterone, which among other things controls the development of the prostate gland. In males androgens are made in the testis and adrenal gland. Prostate cancer is testosterone-sensitive, and this can accelerate the cancer cell growth. Anti-androgen drugs block androgen hormones, in this case testosterone, which will result in slowing down or stopping prostate cancer cell growth. Bicalutamide is an example of anti-androgen.

Progestogens

Oestrogen and progesterone affect the growth and activity of the endometrium and are the hormones responsible for the regulation of the menstrual cycle. Oestrogen influences proliferation of epithelial cells within the endometrium while progesterone constrains cell growth and causes cell differentiation. Endometrial cancers are often ER+, and which means they bind to oestrogen which promotes endometrial cancer cell growth.

The use of progesterone drugs to treat endometrial cancer works by opposing oestrogen-driven cell growth, which results in shrinking the tumour. Medroxyprogesterone acetate is an example of a progesterone.

Side Effects of Hormone Therapy

Each individual hormone treatment has its own side effect profile. Table 9.6 shows the most common general side effects for hormone therapy, and these are similar to the general side effects of traditional cytotoxic agents and menopause symptoms for women and what could be termed a pseudo-menopause for men.

Table 9.6 General side effects of hormone therapy

- Fatigue
- Nausea & vomiting
- Constipation and diarrhoea
- Menopausal symptoms
- Muscle and bone changes
- Hair and bone thinning
- Headaches
- Mood changes and memory problems
- Erectile dysfunction
- Breast tenderness
- Weight gain
- Tumour flare pain

Stop and Think ...

Describe how you would explain to a new nurse how hormone therapies work.

Supportive Therapy

Supportive therapies are not aimed at treating the cancer but are therapies that may make other treatment more effective or manage symptoms caused by disease and/or cancer treatment.

Growth Factors for Blood Cells

We have covered growth factors previously in this chapter in relation to growth factor inhibitors as a treatment for cancer. Growth factors for blood cells are used as supportive therapies.

Earlier in this chapter we mentioned that different growth factors instruct the growth of distinct types of cells, such as endothelial cells, vascular cells, red blood cells and white blood cells. Manufactured growth factors are used to stimulate the bone marrow to make certain types of blood cells when treatment-induced bone marrow suppression occurs.

Granulocyte Colony-Stimulating Factor (G-CSF)

G-CSF is a man-made growth factor that stimulates the growth of erythrocytes, megakaryocytes neutrophils and monocyte macrophages cell lines. These cells have the GCSF receptors on their surface so when G-CSF is administered it will target these receptors to signal cells in this lineage to grow and divide. G-CSF is used as a supportive therapy, particularly for chemotherapy-induced neutropenia to target the cell line growth for this deficiency.

In solid tumours, G-CSF may be given prophylactically to help boost the bone marrow before treatment in making these cells, as there is a high chance that treatment will cause bone marrow suppression particularly in this cell lineage. G-CSF may also be given to treat chemotherapy-induced bone marrow depression, and neutropenia which

Table 9.7 Side effects of GCSF

- Bone pain
- Headaches
- Thrombocytopenia
- Anaemia
- Nausea
- Diarrhoea
- Spleen abnormalities

Table 9.8 Side effects of erythropoietin

- Headache
- Hypertension
- Peripheral oedema
- Skin reactions
- Embolism
- Thrombosis

may prevent treatment being deferred or stopped. Lenograstim is an example of a G-CSF. Table 9.7 lists the common side effects of GCSF.

Erythropoietin

Erythropoietin is a growth factor that stimulates the bone marrow to turn proerythroblasts (immature red blood cells) into mature erythrocytes (red blood cells). Man-made erythropoietin is used as a supportive therapy, particularly for chemotherapy-induced anaemia to target the cell line growth for the deficiency. Although the usual treatment for anaemia is a blood transfusion, the use of man-made erythropoietin in this case can be especially useful to treat anaemia in patients receiving chemotherapy to limit the number of blood transfusions for this group of patients or in cases where a blood transfusion is not suitable. Epoetin alfa is an example of erythropoietin. Table 9.8 lists common side effects of erythropoietin.

Bisphosphonates

Bisphosphonates are drugs that slow down or prevent bone damage. They do this by targeting areas of higher bone turnover. The drug is absorbed by osteoclast cells, which are the cells involved in breaking down old or damaged bone, and slows down the osteoclast cell activity resulting in inhibiting or stopping further bone damage.

Myeloma and cancer that has metastasised to bones cause direct damage to bone which initiates the release of cytokines and growth factors which interfere with the normal process of bone shaping. These stimulate the osteoclast cells to become over-active, and lead to further break down of bone. This results in bones becoming very thin and weak which cause bone pain. The breakdown of bone by the osteoclasts also releases calcium into the blood stream leading to hypercalcaemia. The use of bisphosphonates

Table 9.9 Side effects of bisphosphonates

- Flu like symptoms
- Hypercalcaemia
- Bone and joint pain
- Altered bowel habits
- Fatigue
- Nausea
- Renal damage
- Osteonecrosis of the jaw
- Oesophagitis

as a supportive treatment in myeloma and metastatic bone cancer is to prevent further bone damage, pain control and treat hypercalcaemia. Pamidronate is an example of a bisphosphonate.

General Side Effects of Bisphosphonates

Table 9.9 shows the general side effects from bisphosphonates; there are some specific side effects such as osteonecrosis of the jaw and oesophagitis and more general side effects. These are very similar to the side effect profile of traditional cytotoxic chemotherapy, targeted therapies and hormone treatment. It is important to recognise this, as even though supportive therapies are designed to help support or manage symptoms caused by disease and/or cancer treatment, they can cause further overlapping toxicities for a patient.

Other Supportive Therapies

It is worth noting that many other supportive therapies are used for a patient receiving SACT, such as blood products, platelets and steroids, too many to explore in this chapter. The side effect profile of each of these therapies should also be considered, when used alongside other treatments.

Summary

In this chapter we have included the other therapies used alongside SACT either as treatment for disease or as supportive therapy, and the general side effects of these therapies. It is important to consider that for a person receiving SACT it is not only traditional cytotoxic drugs they are receiving but also multiple action therapies. This is why the term 'chemotherapy' is not an exact description, and the term 'SACT' is now used.

With the addition of other therapies being used to treat cancer comes additional side effects. It is important to be aware of toxicities of the agents being administered including overlapping toxicities, how to identify, assess and manage them.

References

Casati, L., Ciceri, S., Maggi, R. and Bottai, D. (2023) Physiological and pharmacological overview of the gonadotropin releasing hormone. *Biochemical Pharmacology,* 212, p. 115553.

Rose, M. et al. (2020) PARP inhibitors: Clinical relevance, mechanisms of action and tumor resistance. *Frontiers in Cell And Developmental Biology*. [Online] 8564601.

Simons, A. and Cutler, T. (2013) 'Chemotherapy and monoclonal antibodies', in Brown, M. and Cutler, T. (eds) *Haematology nursing*. Oxford: Wiley. p. 281.

Vickers, E. (2025) 'Monoclonal antibodies and small molecules as cancer treatments', in Brown, M. and Cutler, T. (eds) *A beginner's guide to targeted cancer treatments and cancer immunotherapy*. 2nd edition. Sussex: Wiley.

CHAPTER 10

Routes and Place of SACT Delivery

Alison Simons

Introduction

SACT can be delivered within a variety of settings and via different routes. In the first part of this chapter, we will be investigating the most common routes of SACT delivery. We will be discovering the different settings where SACT can be administered in the final part of the chapter.

Routes of SACT Delivery

SACT can be delivered via several routes. Regardless of the route the aim is for SACT to be absorbed systemically or locally and the specific type of SACT agent then works on a cellular level as outlined in Chapter 2. Some routes are more common than others and some SACT agents are only available in a particular form. Therefore only specific cancer regimens will use certain routes of delivery. The use of combination SACT regimens may also mean a patient could receive SACT in a variety of delivery routes. As with any SACT administration, the side effects of treatment must be discussed and information provided on how and when to contact for advice (see Chapter 6). Health and safety measures must be considered (see Chapter 5), and specific measures for particular routes of administration should be observed.

Oral

Oral SACT is defined as SACT taken by mouth and swallowed; this is usually in the form of tablets or capsules but could also be in elixir form. Oral SACT is absorbed into the blood via the gastrointestinal tract, and systemically uptaken. Very often patients self-administer oral SACT at home, so it is vital that patients and caregivers are provided with clear instruction on how and when to take their medication. There may be specific advice for example to take with food, or without food and there could be specific food or drinks to avoid whilst taking oral SACT. It is advisable that oral SACT is swallowed

 DOI: 10.4324/9781003516477-10

with plenty of water to avoid irritation of the mucosa. It is important to mention here that a patient who can no longer tolerate their oral SACT (for example if they are experiencing nausea and vomiting) must be advised to seek support from their oncology team, as this will impact treatment efficacy and outcomes. An alternative route to receive this SACT could be required.

Health and safety precautions still need to be considered as outlined in Chapter 5 (see patient and caregiver safety: SACT tablets or capsules at home). It is preferable that tablets or capsules are not broken or crushed as this increases the risk of accidental exposure and could impede the efficacy of the drug.

Intramuscular (IM) and Subcutaneous (SC)

IM SACT is defined as SACT that is administered into the muscle, and SC SACT is administered under the skin into subcutaneous tissue. IM injections are usually administered in the upper outer quadrant of the buttocks, in the upper thigh or upper arm. While SC injections tend to be in the abdomen, thigh and upper arm, the SACT agent is absorbed via the muscle or skin and taken up systemically. Local policy regarding administration for drugs via these routes should be followed, and the Z track technique for IM administration is advised to minimise risk of exposure and irritation of local tissues and to improve accuracy of delivery into the muscle (Wilkes, 2018) (Figure 10.1). SC SACT can be self-administered at home by the patient, therefore appropriate advice and information must be provided. Particular attention to health and safety measures should be observed as needles are an open source, increasing the risk of accidental exposure and needlestick injuries. Rotation of injection sites, particular with SC injections is important to reduce irritation and discomfort, which may also impact absorption. Injections may cause stinging and minor aches for patients; these tend to be mild and short-lived.

Intravenous (IV)

IV SACT delivery is the most common route of administration, when SACT agents are administered directly into the vein and are rapidly absorbed systemically. Venous access is discussed in Chapter 3. The types of venous access devices are:

- Peripheral cannula
- Central venous access device (CVAD)
- Peripherally inserted central venous catheter (PICC)
- Implantable port

How IV treatment is delivered is dependent on the type of venous access, the SACT agent, dosage and regimen. For example, via IV bolus injection, where a single drug is administered over a short period of time, generally 1–30 minutes by a syringe or short infusion. Continuous intravenous infusion (IVI) is the most common IV SACT delivery. This is a method of continuous administration of fluids including SACT and other drugs, over a longer period. This is an effective delivery mode for combination SACT regimens administering different SACT agents, antiemetics and other drugs sequentially. A continuous IVI can be used via all venous access devices and reduces the number of

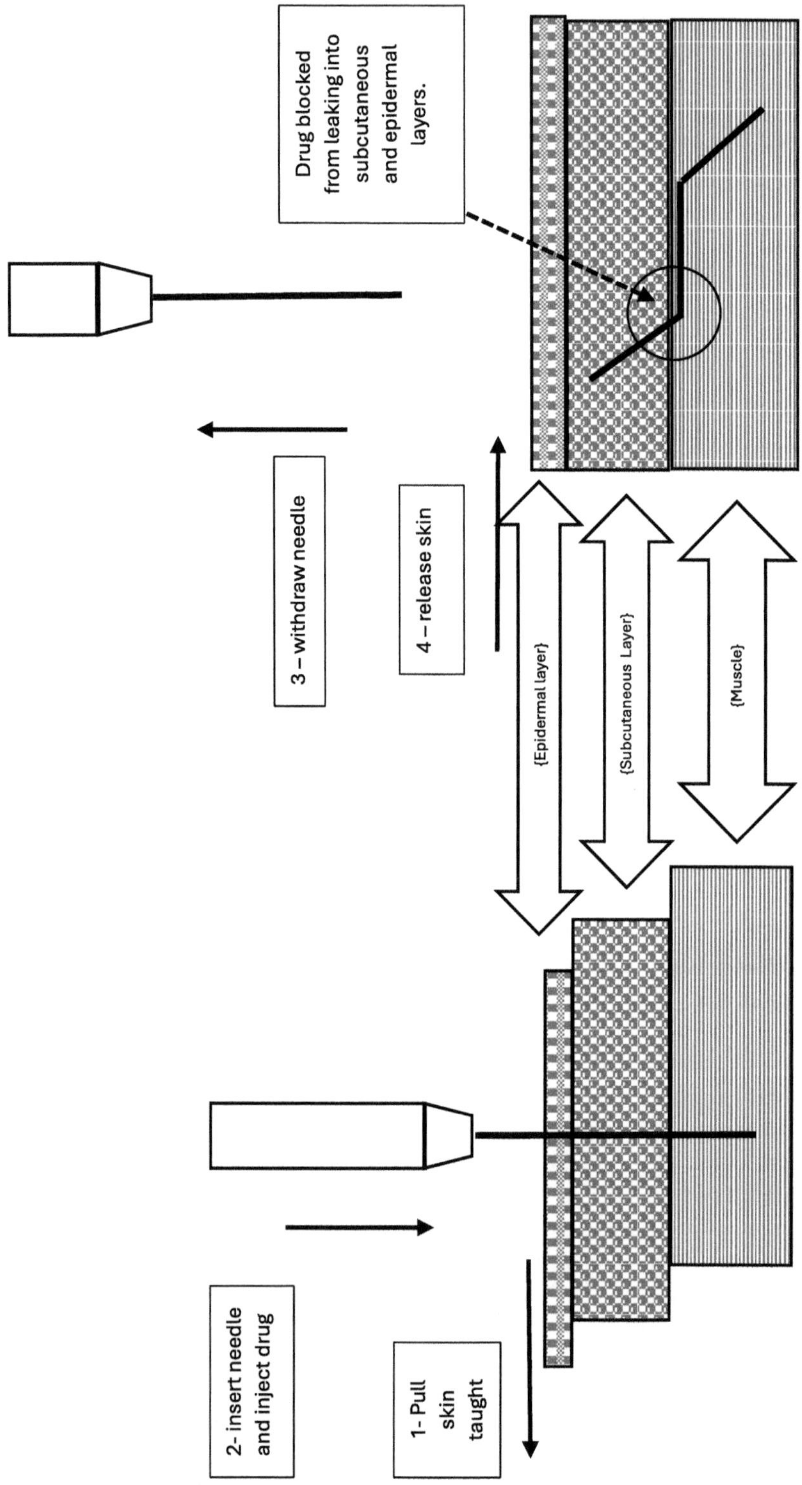

Figure 10.1 Z track IM injection technique

times a device needs to be accessed during longer treatment. This can reduce infection risk and occupational exposure (particularly if using a CSTD as discussed in Chapter 5) and in some cases help preserve venous access. Continuous IVI often use volumetric pumps (VP) to help deliver treatment rather than via gravity-giving sets, as VPs facilitate accurate delivery of drugs over the prescribed rate. However, this is dependent on the accuracy of the SACT practitioner programming the VP. Volumetric pumps are sensitive to occlusions and air, alerting users to this via an alarm and can potentially prevent occlusions due to the constant infusion pressure. Ambulatory pumps can also be used to deliver IV SACT. These are pumps that are designed to be wearable and portable and are used for specific SACT agents to be delivered over several days but can only be used if a CVAD or PICC is in place. Patients will go home wearing these pumps, therefore, advice and information for the patient and their caregivers is vital. The ambulatory pump will need disconnecting after the prescribed time, either by the administering unit or in some cases via district nurse services.

Although IV SACT is the most common and effective way of delivering treatment it is not without challenges. SACT nurses must be aware of the considerations when administering IV SACT and when inserting, accessing and utilising venous devices. For example, extravasation is an emergency where swift appropriate action is required. To ensure safe IV SACT delivery SACT nurses must have knowledge on prevention, assessment, recognition and management of extravasation. This is covered in detail in Chapter 3.

Stop and Think …

How would you explain the common routes of SACT delivery to a member of staff who is new to SACT administration?

Topical

Topical SACT is where treatment is administered in the form of a cream or ointment. Small doses of SACT can be delivered locally to the skin for some skin cancers. This aims to treat cancer cells directly by delivering SACT to the cancer cells, where it is absorbed. Topical SACT will cause skin cancer cells to be destroyed and initially makes the lesion look and feel worse, but this is often a sign that treatment is working. Topical SACT is self-administered by patients or caregivers and strict guidance and information must be provided. Topical treatments lack accuracy in administration and dosage, under dosage of SACT affects efficacy of treatment and overdosing can result in exacerbation of side effects. As topical SACT is applied to the skin, it can be difficult to apply this accurately and if normal skin is included within the delivery zone, damage will be caused, resulting in redness, soreness and blistering of the skin. Repeated long-term treatment of normal skin cells can cause sloughing and weeping and could increase the risk of these cells becoming mutated and malignant. Very often skin cancers occur on the face so this mode of treatment can cause the skin to become unsightly and obvious, impacting self-image, confidence and mood. Health and safety measures for topical SACT are important; administration should not be undertaken without wearing gloves, handwashing and storage of the cream should be observed.

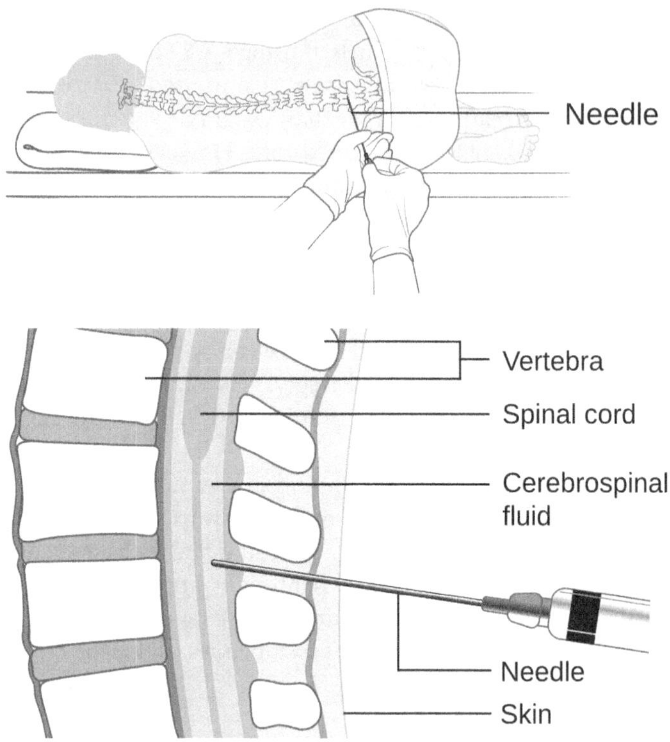

Figure 10.2 Lumbar puncture procedure

Intrathecal (IT)

IT SACT is used to treat cancers that could spread to cerebrospinal fluid (CSF) (a colourless fluid that bathes the spinal cord), such as acute lymphoblastic leukaemia (ALL). IT SACT is injected directly into the CSF via the intrathecal space. Access to the intrathecal space and the CSF is achieved by a lumbar puncture procedure. This procedure involves a needle being inserted between the lumbar vertebrae (L4 and L5) using local anaesthetic (see Figure 10.2).

Once access to the CSF is confirmed, IT SACT can be administered. The use of an Ommaya reservoir can be considered for frequent IT SACT and may be preferred for administration within paediatric patients. This is a reservoir catheter system that is inserted under the scalp via surgery. The catheter enters the ventricles of the brain, allowing direct access to CSF.

IT SACT is considered a high-risk procedure due to the nature of the drugs used and the challenges of the administration process. Following several incidents worldwide involving errors where the incorrect drug was administered intrathecally rather than IV, which resulted in paralysis or death, very strict national guidance was published (Department of Health, 2008). **Only** practitioners that are recorded on the specialist IT register (designated personnel who have been trained and authorised as competent) are permitted to prescribe, dispense, issue, check, administer or assist with this procedure. Other restrictions in place are designated administration areas, strict annual training and competence reviews and regular audits. Current and approved local protocols must be available and read by all staff directly and indirectly involved in any aspect of IT SACT.

Intravesical

Intravesical SACT is used to treat non-muscle invasive bladder cancer and is administered directly into the bladder via a urinary catheter, and the bladder cells take up the SACT drugs. Following insertion of the catheter and administration of SACT, the catheter may be removed. If the catheter is removed, the patient is requested not to urinate for 2 hours. This is not possible for some patients, so this would require leaving the catheter in situ and clamping off the catheter for a prescribed time. This allows the SACT to bathe the endothelial bladder lining and be absorbed, and to ensure the whole bladder lining is treated, the patient needs to change position regularly, for example, from prone to supine. After the prescribed time, the patient may void urine. In some cases, patients may be able to return home once the SACT has been administered and the catheter removed and instructed to void urine after the prescribed time. Ideally, the catheter will have been removed as the act of voiding urine will bathe the urethra, but if the catheter remains in situ it is unclamped to drain the urine and the catheter is removed. The removal and disposal of the catheter and full urine bag containing SACT poses a health and safety risk, as a catheter is in an open source, and splashback is likely. Therefore, attention to safe handling precautions is vital and consideration of wearing eye protection is advised.

Less Common Routes of Administration

Intraperitoneal

Intraperitoneal SACT is when SACT is administered into the peritoneal cavity. This is used to treat cancers within the peritoneal cavity such as ovarian cancer. A drain is inserted into the peritoneal cavity via the abdomen and SACT is administered with the aim of bathing the peritoneal cavity with SACT, which is absorbed systemically. More recently, hyperthermic intraperitoneal chemotherapy (HIPEC) is also being used to treat these cancers. This delivery is undertaken directly following the resection of a cancer. Once the cancer has been removed under general anaesthetic, warmed SACT (to prevent the patient going into shock and to improve the efficacy of SACT) is put into the peritoneal cavity via a drain. The SACT stays within the patient for a prescribed time and then removed at the end of the surgery. Health and safety measures when handling SACT during this process is vital.

Intrapleural

Intrapleural SACT is where SACT is administered into the pleural cavity, which is the space between the pleural membrane and the lung. This is often used for treating lung cancer or cancers that have metastasised to the lung, which can often cause pleural effusion, a build-up of the pleuritic fluid due to cancers blocking fluid from draining. Intrapleural SACT is often administered following drainage of a pleural effusion (pleuritic tap). A catheter is inserted into the pleural cavity (pleuritic space) via the chest, and pleural fluid is drained off; this creates a space for the SACT to be administered. The aim is to bathe the pleura with SACT to treat any cancerous cells, so ideally the patient should change their position regularly to ensure all the cavity is treated. This can be problematic for some patients, as due to their disease, they are often short of breath and cannot tolerate lying flat, particularly supine. Pleuritic pain and inflammation can be experienced, but is usually short-lived.

Isolated Limb Perfusion (ILP)

ILP is used to treat recurring melanoma in a limb. This is where SACT is administered directly into a leg or arm, aiming for limb salvage. The limb being treated is isolated from the rest of the body so that SACT can be administered solely to that area to minimise systemic uptake. The procedure is given under general anaesthetic and is only suitable for some patients, well enough to tolerate the procedure. The major blood vessels to the limb being treated are located and cannulated, and a tourniquet is applied to the top of the limb. The cannula is connected to two catheters, which are connected to a perfusion or bypass machine. This recreates the blood circulation to maintain the blood flow around the limb. SACT and oxygen are administered into the blood supply as it passes through the perfusion/bypass machine for a prescribed time (see Figure 10.3).

Due to the limb being isolated during treatment, the rest of the body will not receive SACT. Therefore, a high dose can be administered with potential minimal systemic side effects experienced. However, this procedure is not without risk, for example, infection, thrombosis, nerve damage and lymphoedema. This procedure can be uncomfortable and vein irritation and inflammation can occur.

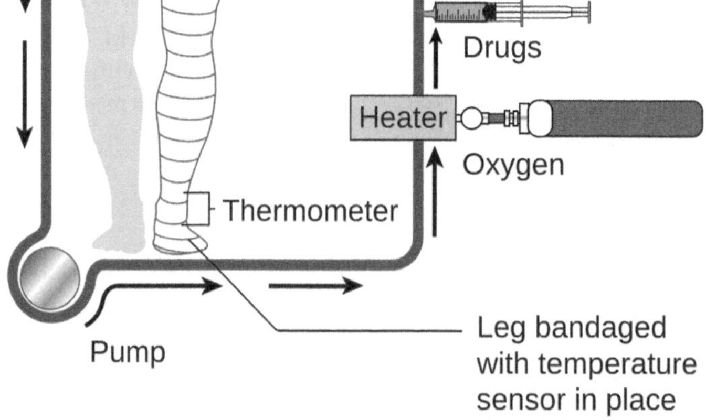

Figure 10.3 Isolated limb perfusion bypass circuit

Isolated limb infusion (ILI) may be used instead of ILP in some cases. This is where a pump is not used, no oxygen is added to SACT, and the prescribed time of infusion is reduced.

Intra-Arterial

This is where SACT is administered into the arteries surrounding the cancer (Lister and Dougherty, 2018). The procedure involves cannulation of the artery under local anaesthetic. This mode of delivery allows high-dose SACT to be administered directly to the cancer and minimises systemic delivery. Intra-arterial SACT is commonly used to treat primary liver disease, liver metastases and retinoblastomas and is only offered in specialised units and might not be widely available to all patients.

Embolisation

TRANS-ARTERIAL EMBOLISATION (TAE)

Embolisation refers to the procedure that blocks the blood supply to a cancer. This is done by injecting gel or beads via the femoral artery into the liver arterial supply. TAE is used to treat contained hepatocellular carcinomas that cannot be surgically resected, and less commonly for secondary liver cancer from a neuroendocrine cancer (NET). The aim of embolisation is to reduce the liver cancer's oxygen and nutrient supply to shrink the cancer size and prevent growth. This may mean that the cancer would be small enough for surgical resection. TAE is performed within the radiology department to ensure accuracy of delivery.

TRANS-ARTERIAL CHEMOEMBOLISATION (TACE)

TACE refers to the procedure when SACT drugs are administered via the femoral artery into the liver arterial supply, followed by administration of gel or beads to block the blood supply (TAE). TACE is used to treat contained hepatocellular carcinomas that cannot be surgically resected and less commonly for secondary liver cancer from bowel cancer or NET. It is performed within the radiology department to ensure accuracy of delivery. In some cases, drug-eluting beads (DEB) are used, which gradually release SACT whilst blocking the blood vessels (DEB-TACE).

Places of SACT Delivery

As SACT drugs and regimens have advanced, how and where this treatment is given has also evolved. Initially, patients were only able to receive treatment on a cancer ward as an inpatient or a chemotherapy unit. SACT can now be administered in a variety of settings based on the specific treatment regimen and person-centred care. Whichever setting SACT is administered within, it must be undertaken by personnel who are trained and competent in caring for patients receiving SACT treatment. Robust pre-treatment assessment, identification and management of adverse effects and emergencies must be carried out, and health and safety measures must be strictly observed. Medical cover to offer advice and support when required should be readily available. All settings are responsible for providing treatment information, including contact details of when and who to contact if they experience side effects or feel unwell.

Oncology Inpatient

Some SACT regimens still require treatment to be administered in a controlled way over a few days, and this would require patients to be hospital inpatients. This tends to be for treatment requiring prolonged pre- and post-treatment hydration due to the type of drugs being used, for example, those that are highly nephrotoxic, and when multi-SACT agents are being administered sequentially. Intensive SACT regimens as part of the preconditioning workup for stem cell transplantation will also require a prolonged hospital stay. Inpatient treatment can often be required for patients at high risk of reactions and therefore need close continuous monitoring. Some SACT regimens require the first course of treatment to be administered as an inpatient to assess toleration. Following assessment, subsequent treatment may be able to be administered in an outpatient setting.

Chemotherapy Day Unit or Ambulatory Unit (Outpatient)

Intravenous SACT (bolus or continuous infusion) is often administered in a chemotherapy day or ambulatory unit. These outpatient units are only open for a specific number of hours and do not have the facilities or are staffed to offer overnight stays for patients. For this reason, these units will only administer treatment that is delivered over a few hours, and this is usually done in a chair rather than a bed. A family member or friend can accompany and stay with the patient for the duration of treatment. Specialist SACT nurses, medics and pharmacists are available to review if patients are fit for treatment before prescribing and administering treatment. Day units facilitate venous access, blood sampling, regular monitoring of patients during administration, information provision for patients and their carers and discharge coordination, for example, providing medication to be taken at home, such as antiemetics.

Home

SACT may be administered in a patient's home in certain circumstances, for example, when a patient is taking SACT orally, topically, intramuscularly, subcutaneously or receiving SACT via a continuous infusion via an ambulatory pump (see routes of SACT delivery). In some cases, a home care SACT nurse service may be appropriate and available to administer SACT to patients within their own home. Receiving treatment at home may be a more patient-centred approach, and may alleviate travelling and associated costs and concerns, and provide a more relaxed environment for patients. However isolation and the opportunity to talk with other people with cancer receiving SACT is missed, which could be beneficial for some patients. The health and safety of other household members must be considered, including the action to take to minimise accidental exposure and management of a spillage in the home (see Chapter 5). Some patients may be able to continue working during treatment. In some cases, such as for private healthcare providers, SACT could also be delivered at a person's workplace, where this has been risk-assessed as safe and appropriate to do so.

Other Settings

In some cases, SACT may be administered in other settings, for example, in radiology departments (see embolisation), operating theatres (see hyperthermic intraperitoneal chemotherapy and isolated limb perfusion), and potentially non-oncological settings (see intravesical and intraperitoneal). It is important to note that SACT is also administered to treat non-malignant conditions, for example, autoimmune diseases (such as lupus, rheumatoid arthritis and ulcerative colitis), sickle cell anaemia and ectopic pregnancy. In these cases, SACT will be delivered within settings that are outside of the oncology field. It is particularly important that within settings that administer SACT less frequently and in fewer patients than a specialised SACT treatment administration setting, fitness for treatment is assessed robustly. SACT practitioners must have knowledge of the agents they are administering in terms of action, side effects, emergencies, health and safety.

Stop and Think ...

What might be the challenges that could be faced in the delivery of SACT in each of the different settings?

Summary

This chapter has explored the different routes of SACT delivery and the different settings for SACT administration. The selection of route and setting must be considered carefully to ensure that treatment is delivered safely, and a person-centred approach is adopted. Regardless of how and where a person receives SACT, the following must be observed: information provision (including side effects and who to contact if they become unwell) and health and safety. In addition, practitioners involved in SACT treatment in each setting and via each route must be competently trained in the handling, administration, caring for patients receiving SACT and managing side effects or emergencies.

References

Department of Health (2008) *HSC 2008/01: Updated national guidance on the safe administration of intrathecal chemotherapy*. London: Department of Health. Available online https://webarchive.nationalarchives.gov.uk/ukgwa/20130104175622/http:/www.dh.gov.uk/en/Publicationsandstatistics/Lettersandcirculars/Healthservicecirculars/DH_086870 Accessed on 18 March 2026

Lister, S. and Dougherty, L. (2018) 'Administration of systemic anticancer therapies', in Sara L. (ed). *The royal marsden manual of cancer nursing procedures*. United Kingdom: Wiley. p. 333.

Wilkes, G.M. (2018) 'Chemotherapy: Principles of administration', in Yarbo, C.H., Wujcik, D. and Holmes Gobel, B. (eds) *Cancer nursing principles and practice*. 8th edition. Burlington, MA: Jones and Barlett Learning, Chapter 15, p. 441.

CHAPTER 11

Beyond physical burden, psychological and psychosocial burden of SACT

Emma Filby

Introduction

SACT is a key part of modern cancer treatment. However, the impact goes beyond the physical effects of the disease and treatment itself. Patients often experience psychological and psychosocial challenges, which can affect their well-being, treatment experience and outcomes. These needs can be overlooked in busy clinical environments as the focus is often on treatment delivery. Understanding the difference between psychological and psychosocial needs and how they can overlap is important when providing holistic cancer care. Tools such as the holistic needs assessment (HNA) can help identify and address concerns, which supports a personalised and coordinated approach to care. This chapter will explore these concepts in relation to SACT and aims to support healthcare practitioners to recognise and respond to the wider needs of the patient throughout their treatment pathway.

Psychological and Psychosocial Impact of Cancer

A cancer diagnosis presents significant challenges for patients, not only physically, but also psychologically and psychosocially. These challenges are not limited to the diagnosis of cancer but are also experienced during the receipt of cancer treatments and their side effects. For some patients, the impact goes well beyond the end of treatment and into survivorship, leading to long-lasting effects on mental health and quality of life. As cancer survival rates continue to improve, there is a comparable increase in the number of people living with psychological and psychosocial effects following cancer and its treatment.

Often, psychological and psychosocial concepts in healthcare are misunderstood and used interchangeably, even though they refer to distinct aspects of a patient's well-being as outlined in seminal work by Engel (1977) and Gater et al. (1991). It is important to recognise these differences to support patient well-being and care outcomes more appropriately, while also recognising that one aspect may influence the other. This is

DOI: 10.4324/9781003516477-11

why healthcare practitioners must build rapport with patients to foster the therapeutic relationship, to improve concordance with care and outcomes (Beach et al., 2016).

Psychological

The term psychological refers to the mental or emotional well-being of an individual, such as anxiety, depression, fear or adjustment difficulties. These issues can arise at any point within a cancer patient's pathway and can be amplified if a patient has a pre-existing mental health condition. Patients can suffer from these difficulties to different degrees, for example, mild anxiety or attempts at suicide. During SACT administration, anxiety or fear are commonly anticipated and sometimes observed. However, more subtle issues like adjustment difficulties or depression are largely overlooked due to the fast pace and high acuity of SACT unit environments. Conversely, healthcare practitioners practising in inpatient areas are more likely to detect the more subtle psychological changes due to the time spent with the patient and the therapeutic relationships built between both the patient and their family.

Psychosocial

Psychosocial concerns reflect a person within their wider context, including their family life, home environment, employment, social networks and practical circumstances. Rather than focusing solely on mental well-being, psychosocial factors relate to how a diagnosis and or the treatment may present external challenges that may be difficult for patients to overcome. For example, a patient undergoing treatment may be struggling with attending appointments due to financial burden, as a direct result of not being able to work due to the debilitating side effects of SACT. The psychosocial impact of cancer treatment is therefore not isolated to the psychological well-being of a patient; it is considered the relationship between social conditions and mental health.

Stop and Think …

Can you explain the difference between psychological and psychosocial to a new member of staff or a patient?

Personalised Care

Due to the impact cancer has on an individual, care must promote the principles of "Getting it Right First Time" (GIRFT) (Getting it Right First Time, 2021). The national cancer plan (Department of Health and Social Care and NHS England, 2026) emphasises that every cancer patient should receive a personalised assessment of need to develop an individualised care plan. This approach focuses on a patient's values, personal priorities and personal circumstances, instead of following a standardised care pathway, recognising the importance of addressing psychological and psychosocial needs. Supporting patient-led decision-making promotes concordance and self-management, providing a real reflection of person-centred care (NHS England, 2019).

To meet the objectives of the cancer plan (Department of Health and Social Care and NHS England, 2026), cancer centres across the United Kingdom must focus on what matters most to the patient. This will be achieved using an enhanced holistic needs assessment (HNA) designed to incorporate health and well-being support, treatment summaries and cancer care reviews following completion of treatment. This approach goes beyond person-centred care; it seeks to ensure the care is also coordinated across hospital, primary care and community settings, i.e. the neighbourhood as defined in the cancer plan. This approach focuses on supporting the person holistically across the cancer pathway, ensuring all needs are identified and addressed through a coordinated multidisciplinary approach. For SACT practitioners, personalised care means assessments are beyond the physiological assessment, but also the psychological and psychosocial impact of cancer and SACT. However, it is not for the SACT practitioner to manage these concerns; it is about facilitating holistic conversations, supporting self-management through signposting, education and appropriate referrals to other services and specialist professionals.

Holistic Needs Assessment (HNA)

The HNA is an assessment completed by the patient, with outcomes discussed with a member of the cancer healthcare team. It considers not only the physical aspects of diagnosis and treatment, but also the psychological and psychosocial needs of the individual. The HNA identifies and prioritises concerns as defined by the patient, focusing on what matters most to them. However, the effectiveness of the HNA is dependent on how consistently and meaningfully it is implemented, as well as how thoroughly and honestly the patient completes it. If it is used as a 'tick box' exercise, there is a risk that patients' concerns are not fully explored or acted upon, which limits the impact on patient outcomes.

The healthcare practitioner can address priority concerns through education, pharmacological and non-pharmacological interventions, as well as signposting or referrals to other services, such as counselling, help with finance, help with meals, or support groups. Concerns identified through the HNA are often interrelated, resulting in overlapping psychological and psychosocial challenges. Therefore, addressing a patient's priority concerns can often simultaneously alleviate related issues, making them feel more manageable for the patient and contributing to an improvement in overall quality of life. See Table 11.1 for examples of how concerns identified through the HNA can be categorised as either psychological or psychosocial, and how they may overlap.

Completing the HNA can feel time-consuming, especially in busy SACT environments and this can create a challenge between meeting time demands and providing high-quality holistic care. As a result, psychological and psychosocial support may be overlooked or deprioritised over physical treatment delivery. However, the HNA is recommended at key points along the patient pathway, at diagnosis, during treatment and after treatment is finished. In many organisations the HNA is completed by a designated member of the healthcare team rather than the SACT practitioner. There is also variation in how the HNA is carried out and followed up, which may lead to differences in patient experience and access to support. Despite this, the SACT practitioner remains well placed to recognise and address psychological and psychosocial concerns during routine clinical interactions. A SACT practitioner may identify a holistic concern at the point of toxicity screening through therapeutic conversations. This

Table 11.1 Distinguishment between psychosocial and psychological concerns through the Holistic Needs Assessment and how concerns can overlap

HNA Concern	*Psychological issues*	*Psychosocial issues*	*Potential overlap*
Emotional well-being	• Treatment anxiety • Fear of recurrence • Depression • Adjustment difficulties	• Reduced social engagement • Withdrawal from support networks	Emotional distress may lead to social withdrawal or reduced engagement with family and friends. The reduced engagement can lead to depression or adjustment difficulties
Family and relationships	• Feelings of guilt or burden • Worry about family members	• Relationship strain • Sexual intimacy • Change in family role • Caregiving responsibilities	Emotional distress may affect communication within relationships or family dynamics. The lack of communication may heighten worry or feelings of guilt
Work and finances	• Stress or anxiety about job security, or financial pressures	• Loss of employment • Reduced income • Financial Hardship	Financial strain can increase anxiety. Increased risk of depression or emotional distress due to job security.
Daily living and independence	• Loss of confidence • Reduced self esteem • Frustration due to disease or side effects	• Loss of independence • Difficulty with practical elements (washing and dressing)	Loss of independence can cause issues with identity, confidence and emotional well-being. In addition, it can reinforce frustration based on the disease or side effects.
Social support	• Feelings of loneliness or isolation	• Reduced ability to be involved in social networks	Loneliness can lead to disengagement; disengagement can reinforce loneliness and isolation
Spiritual concerns	• Fear of death • Questioning beliefs	• Reduced ability to be involved in faith communities or spiritual practices	Inability to engage can reinforce fears and questioning.
SACT experience	• Fear of treatment • Anxiety over side effects	• Childcare or work disruption • Travel issues	Practical issues can heighten treatment related fear and anxiety

could trigger a formal HNA through organisational process, or prompt action, such as providing simple evidence-based advice, signposting, or appropriate referral, as a result, improving a patient's quality of life, SACT experience and personalised care planning.

Patients can feel completely overwhelmed by the psychological and psychosocial burden associated with SACT, which can influence treatment agreement decisions, or mean they cannot proceed with treatment as planned. The HNA can reveal vital information that could change the course of a patient's treatment. Their psychological and psychosocial needs may need to be addressed before SACT can be administered safely, for example, if they are the main carer of a dependent. In such cases, a patient's circumstances may require a temporary deferral of treatment to ensure they are adequately supported, both psychologically and psychosocially, before continuation. This has the potential to lead to dishonesty through fear of the deferral of treatment.

Stop and Think ...

Think of some of your patients, how did they feel before they started SACT? Which were psychological? and which were psychosocial?

Psychological and Psychosocial Impact of Common SACT Side Effects

SACT can cause a range of side effects, which vary in severity for each person and can extend beyond the physiological symptoms and affect a person's overall quality of life. As previously discussed, the psychological and psychosocial issues a patient experiences are equally important to address to ensure the patient receives personalised care which is bespoke to their personal needs. Table 11.2 looks at the common SACT side effects and potential impact on a psychological and psychosocial level, with suggestive practical advice and interventions.

Table 11.2 shows some repetition across the side effects, highlighting how addressing one concern may help alleviate other concerns. The guidance is not exhaustive; alternative or additional interventions may be more appropriate depending on the patient's individual circumstances, alongside local and national policy and clinical guidelines and the current evidence-based research. SACT practitioners must consider these factors before offering advice or making referrals, ensuring care is evidence-based, aligned with organisation policy and the principles of beneficence. Equally, patient concerns should not be overlooked or dismissed due to workload pressures or assumptions that another healthcare professional will address them. SACT practitioners have a clear duty of care and failure to recognise and respond to patient needs may compromise the principle of non-maleficence.

Stop and Think ...

How would you support the patient with any psychological and psychosocial concerns? Can you think of self-help strategies, signposting advice or appropriate referrals?

SACT Practitioner Knowledge and Skills

Supporting patients effectively is vital to help maintain quality of life and overall SACT experience, as outlined in the NMC Code (2018); the healthcare practitioner must remain current in their knowledge and key skills.

Table 11.2 SACT side effects impacting psychological and psychosocial well-being

Side effect	*Psychological*	*Psychosocial*	*Practical Guidance*
Nausea & vomiting	• Anticipatory nausea • Anxiety • Depression	• Social Isolation • Financial implications	• Antiemetics review/prescribe • Keep a diary for pattern identification to aid coping strategy • Refer for financial support • Advise on any support groups • Referral to dietician for advice on diet to avoid weight loss and aid recovery from SACT cycles • Referral to counselling services • Practical advice as per organisational policy i.e. avoiding favourite foods
Constipation	• Depression • Self-esteem issues	• Insomnia from discomfort • Social isolation	• Gentle exercise • Review medication and consider laxatives • Advise on any support groups • Increase fluid intake • Refer to a dietician for dietary advice • Practical advice as per organisational policy
Diarrhoea	• Anxiety relating to accidents in public • Depression with chronic diarrhoea	• Public avoidance • Social isolation • Financial implications	• Review medication and consider antidiarrheal medication • Refer for financial support • Advise on any support groups • Referral to dietician for advice on diet • Referral to counselling services • Practical advice as per organisational policy
Anorexia	• Self-esteem issues • Sense of hopelessness • Fear of death • Depression	• Social isolation • Conflict with family over food	• Keeping a food diary, monitoring for patterns • Refer to the dietician for build up supplements and dietary advice • Referral to counselling services • Advise on any support groups • Practical advice as per organisational policy
Fatigue	• Anxiety • Hopelessness • Depression	• Social Isolation • Financial implications • Relationship and family dynamics	• Gentle exercise • Refer to counselling services • Advise on any support groups • Refer for financial support • Practical advice as per organisational policy i.e. sleeping when required, rather than at night

(Continued)

Table 11.2 (Continued)

Side effect	*Psychological*	*Psychosocial*	*Practical Guidance*
Mucositis	• Anxiety • Depression	• Public avoidance • Social isolation	• Encourage oral hygiene as per organisational policy • Consider analgesia where required • Referral to counselling services • Advise on any support groups • Practical advice as per organisational policy i.e. pineapple, ice chips, oral cryotherapy
Neuropathy /Skin reactions	• Anxiety • Depression	• Public avoidance • Social isolation • Financial implications • Relationship and family dynamics	• Advise on any support groups • Referral to counselling services • Practical advice as per organisational policy
Hair loss	• Self esteem • Depression • Loss of identity	• Relationships • Public avoidance • social isolation • Financial implications	• Scalp cooling where appropriate • Wig referrals • Headscarves and hats • Referral to counselling services • Advise on any support groups • Refer for financial support • Practical advice as per organisational policy i.e. cutting hair short, "look good, feel good" initiatives

Skills

Skills such as communication are a large part of delivering SACT care, from gaining informed consent, educating patients around their disease or treatment in a non-jargonistic manner and facilitating complex conversations relating to subjects such as death and dying, or psychological or psychosocial distress caused by cancer and its treatment. Therefore, to facilitate interactions effectively and provide a high standard of person-centred care, advanced communication skills are paramount, not only to allow the conversations to flow more effectively and have a beneficial outcome for the patient, but also to support the healthcare practitioner in what can be challenging conversations.

Knowledge

A SACT practitioner needs to understand the diseases, but also the treatments, their administration processes, side effects and emergency protocols. The SACT practitioner also needs to be familiar with national and local support groups, charities and services available to support the patient holistically. This information needs to be accurate to avoid inaccurate signposting and delaying treatment support. In addition, the SACT practitioner needs to be familiar with local and national policy and standard operating procedures to ensure the correct interventions and advice are offered, for example, knowing how to refer a patient to the dieticians or counselling services. Delays can have a detrimental impact on the patient and their treatment.

Resilience

Personal and professional resilience is an essential skill for SACT practitioners working within increasingly pressurised environments, facing rising workloads with new treatments and reduced staffing. SACT practitioners often develop therapeutic relationships with patients and support them throughout their treatment journey, which can include both positive outcomes and disease progression. This sustained emotional engagement can impact the SACT practitioner, contributing to emotional fatigue. As a result, SACT practitioners are at risk of burnout and compassion fatigue, which may affect both the practitioner's well-being and the quality of patient care delivered. These challenges can lead to increased absenteeism, further exacerbating workforce pressures. As a result, patients may feel reluctant to share their concerns for fear of burdening staff, which can potentially result in unmet psychological and psychosocial needs.

Given the specialist knowledge and skills required within SACT practice, it is vital that practitioners actively engage in strategies to support their own well-being and maintain their resilience. These strategies may include individual approaches such as exercise, hobbies and maintaining a healthy work/life balance. In addition, organisational support is crucial to support SACT practitioners to maintain their mental well-being. Effective leadership should prioritise staff well-being through the provision of clinical supervision, regular team debriefs and opportunities to reflect and celebrate successes.

Summary

In summary, the psychological and psychosocial impact of SACT can be significant, interrelated and at times under-recognised. Delivering effective person-centred coordinated care requires SACT practitioners to proactively identify and address patient concerns through a holistic, collaborative and personalised approach supported by best practice and structured assessment tools. Furthermore, practitioner well-being is integral to the delivery of compassionate care. Supporting personal resilience enables practitioners to sustain the emotional demands of the role and maintain the ability to provide holistic care. Holistic care should be regarded as fundamental rather than optional, with essential early identification and intervention to prevent escalation of unmet needs and optimise patient outcomes.

References

Beach, M.C., Sugarman, J., Johnson, J., et al. (2016) Do patients treated with dignity report higher satisfaction, adherence, and receipt of preventive care? A survey of diverse patients in primary care. *Patient Education and Counseling*, 99(3), pp. 353–360.

Department of Health and Social Care and NHS England (2026) *The National Cancer Plan for England: Delivering world class cancer care*. London: Crown copyright. Accessed: 06 March 2026 [online] via: https://assets.publishing.service.gov.uk/media/699ec931532c9ad91ebbcc64/national-cancer-plan-for-england-delivering-world-class-cancer-care.pdf

Engel, G.L. (1977) The need for a new medical model: A challenge for biomedicine. *Science*, 196(4286), pp. 129–136.

Gater, R., Goldberg, D. and Faragher, B. (1991) Psychosocial factors and medical illness. *British Journal of Psychiatry*, 159, pp. 6–15.
NHS England (2019) *The NHS long term plan*. London: NHS England.
NHS England (2021) *Getting It Right First Time (GIRFT): Programme overview and national reports*. London: NHS England. Available [online] at: www.gettingitrightfirsttime.co.uk Accessed: 06 March 2026.
Nursing and Midwifery Council (NMC) (2018) *The Code: Professional standards of practice and behaviour for nurses, midwives and nursing associates*. London: NMC.

CHAPTER 12

Leadership and Multiprofessional Co-Ordinated Care

Emma Filby

Introduction

Leadership is often seen as a role for senior staff, but in healthcare, leadership can be demonstrated by any professional at any level. In SACT services, effective leadership ensures care is person-centred, safe and coordinated across the disciplines and services. The Nursing and Midwifery Council (NMC, 2018) recognises leadership as a core standard for registered nurses, forming part of pre-registration programmes across the United Kingdom. This chapter provides a deeper understanding of leadership, recognising that leadership is less complex than it first appears and relates to all healthcare professionals across multiple disciplines and services. In addition, it will support the recognition of the importance of leadership in the safe and effective delivery of SACT.

What Is Leadership?

There is no single, set definition of the term leadership. However, many researchers and practitioners have attempted to explain what constitutes good leadership and its importance in delivering safe, high-quality, person-centred care. Aristotle, an ancient Greek philosopher and polymath (384–322BC), suggested, "He who cannot be a good follower cannot be a good leader", which highlights the mutual relationship between leadership and followership. Simon Sinek, an inspirational speaker on business leadership, often explains, "Leadership is not about being in charge. It's about taking care of those in your charge" (Sinek, 2014), suggesting leadership is relational rather than hierarchical. However, Michael West CBE, who has published numerous works on healthcare leadership, focuses on compassionate leadership. Suggesting compassionate leadership is a form of "collective, inclusive leadership grounded in attending, understanding, empathising, and helping, which creates psychological safety and enables individuals and teams to relieve suffering, improve performance, innovation, and quality in health and social care settings". This approach suggests that psychological safety enables

DOI: 10.4324/9781003516477-12

individuals and teams to reduce suffering and improve performance, innovation and quality in healthcare provision (West et al., 2017). The NMC echo West's research when they launched the "Good Leadership means better care" campaign in 2023, highlighting the importance of leadership enabling the delivery of safe, high-quality care. Each of these ideas highlights interesting insights into leadership and can be considered quite influential and inspirational in some situations. Before we look at what all this means and how leadership is utilised to support healthcare practitioners working within SACT services, let's look at what these leadership mean to you.

Stop and Think

What do you think leadership is? Who should be a leader? How do you think leadership supports SACT care delivery?

Leadership Theories

Effective leadership is the foundation of providing safe co-ordinated person-centred care. It is not defined by hierarchy and is not limited to managers or senior staff. Instead, it can be seen in anyone within the team, whether it is the individual taking charge of a shift in a SACT day unit or a SACT practitioner leading a patient's care, meaning leadership is dynamic, situational and shaped by context. Leadership theories help us understand how people lead, the behaviours and characteristics associated with effective leadership and how leadership influences team performance and patient outcomes. By understanding these theories, healthcare professionals can reflect on their own practice, adapt to challenges and contribute to team environments that promote collaboration, innovation and high-quality person-centred care.

In the following sections, we will explore key leadership theories, from historical models such as the Great Man and Trait Theories to contemporary approaches including Behavioural, Transactional, Transformational and Compassionate Leadership. Each theory will provide a different lens through which leadership will be viewed, using a scenario of an extravasation, to support comparison and application of the theories.

The Great Man Theory

In the 19th century, Thomas Carlyle developed the Great Man Theory; his idea was that leaders were born with certain traits naturally giving them the ability to succeed and lead effectively (Carlyle, 1974). He argued that effective leadership was for "great men" of high social status, believing that status naturally brings authority, sound judgement and the ability to maintain order through charm and charisma (Carlyle, 1974). In modern healthcare, this theory holds little credibility due to its lack of scientific evidence. However, elements of the Great Man Theory can still be seen in practice today. Applying this theory to our extravasation scenario, teams may instinctively look to the most senior member of staff to take control of the emergency, reflecting the assumption that leadership is linked to status and authority, rather than capability or behaviour.

Trait Theory

Trait Theory came from the Great Man Theory, moving away from the idea of social status towards specific personal characteristics associated with leadership. Instead of assuming leaders are defined by position or background, it suggests that qualities such as intelligence, integrity, confidence and determination distinguish leaders from others (Northouse, 2022). In the extravasation scenario, the practitioner who appears confident may naturally take charge and the team may follow them. However, confidence does not always equal competence, and quieter individuals may possess equal or greater skill and knowledge. As a result, this leadership trait could lead to assumptions about leadership ability based on perception rather than actual ability and knowledge.

Behavioural Theory

Behavioural Theory represents a significant shift from innate traits to observable actions. Leadership can be learned and demonstrated through behaviours such as clear communication, delegation and decision-making (Northouse, 2022). During an extravasation incident, a practitioner demonstrating behavioural leadership would promptly recognise the situation, raise the alarm for support, delegate tasks appropriately, communicate clearly with the team and provide reassurance to the patient while ensuring the incident is managed according to organisational policy. Leadership here is about what you do rather than who you are; even a junior practitioner can take the lead if they demonstrate the appropriate behaviours and have the right skill set.

Transactional Theory

Transactional leadership is structured and task-focused, meaning leaders will set the goals and expectations of the team, and these goals will be achieved based on reward (Bass and Avolio, 1994). In simple terms, it is about ensuring that the job gets done, standards are met and any issues are addressed promptly. In the extravasation scenario, the practitioner ensures that tasks are completed correctly, roles are clearly defined, and documentation is thorough. This approach supports patient safety, adherence to policy and accountability. Although this achieves results, a purely transactional approach may limit opportunities for team reflection or development. Relying on a task-focused approach can also affect patient experience. The Mid Staffordshire NHS Foundation Trust inquiry highlighted how prioritising targets and processes over human factors contributed to failures in compassionate care (Francis, 2013). This shows that while transactional leadership provides structure and safety, it must be balanced with approaches that support both team and patient well-being.

Transformational Leadership Theory

Transformational Leadership Theory focuses on how leaders influence and motivate others to work towards a shared goal, instead of relying on authority or position (Northouse, 2022). It emphasises the relationship between leaders and their teams,

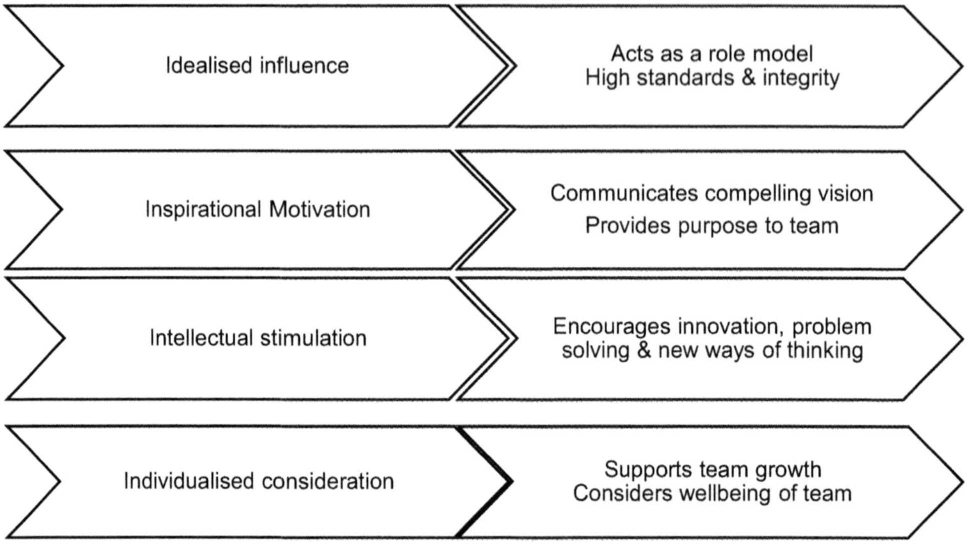

Figure 12.1 Image of diagram outlining transformational leadership characteristics

highlighting how individuals can be supported and challenged to achieve more than expected. The theory is underpinned by four key characteristics: idealised influence, inspirational motivation, intellectual simulation and individualised consideration. These are illustrated in Figure 12.1, which outlines how transformational leadership can be demonstrated in practice.

In SACT practice, a transformational practitioner would not only manage the extravasation but also facilitate reflection, encourage discussion of what went well, and explore areas for improvement with the team. By supporting team learning, transformational leadership fosters confidence, innovation, and collaboration.

Compassionate Theory

Compassionate leadership focuses on empathy, awareness of others' needs, and promoting psychological safety (West et al., 2017). It focuses on leaders' awareness of the experiences and needs of others, it encourages active listening, supportive reactions without judgement and creating a team culture of psychological safety and trust, which leads to positive team well-being. This theory recognises that healthcare environments are emotionally and cognitively demanding, and that effective leadership must include both performance and the well-being of individuals in the team. In SACT services, compassionate leadership is particularly important, as teams are under extreme pressure, managing complex treatments while supporting patients through stressful experiences. In our extravasation scenario, a compassionate practitioner would manage the clinical situation according to policy while also considering the emotional impact on both the patient and colleagues. Reassurance, supportive communication and opportunities for reflection complement transactional and transformational approaches, creating a balance between safety, team motivation and well-being.

Table 12.1 Application of leadership theory in practice

Theory	*How leadership is viewed*	*Practice example: extravasation*
Great man	Status and authority	Team looks to the most senior clinician to take control
Trait	Personal characteristics	Team follows the practitioner who appears most confident
Behavioural	Actions and behaviours	Practitioner leads through clear communication, delegation and safe practice
Transformational	Inspiring and developing others	Practitioner supports team learning and reflection after the event
Transactional	Structure, roles and task-oriented	Practitioner follows protocol, ensuring tasks are completed correctly
Compassionate	Empathy, support and well-being	Practitioner supports the patient and the team emotionally during and after the incident

Leadership Theories Summary

By comparing these theories, it becomes clear that effective leadership in SACT settings requires a combination of situational awareness, structured practice, motivation, development and empathy. While the theories differ in focus, from status, traits and behaviours to motivation and compassion, when used together they provide a practical framework for reflecting on leadership in practice. Table 12.1 provides a summary of how each theory can be applied in practice.

Leadership Styles

Leadership theory explores the principles, frameworks and evidence behind effective leadership, whereas leadership styles focus on how those principles are applied in practice. Styles reflect the behaviours, attitudes and approaches leaders use to guide a team. In this section, we will explore leadership styles commonly seen in healthcare, particularly in SACT settings and consider how different approaches can influence team performance, patient safety and the delivery of person-centred care. However, no one leadership style can be applied to all scenarios; an effective leader will adapt their leadership approach to the given situation.

Authoritarian Leadership

Authoritarian leadership involves setting clear expectations about what needs to be done, when and how, usually without seeking input from anyone in the team. This approach can be highly effective in situations that demand rapid, decisive action, but it can also create tension if overused, as no one likes being told what to do. Let's look at some examples of when authoritarian leadership works and hinders the delivery of person-centred care. Consider a patient having an allergic reaction to SACT, leading to cardiac arrest. An experienced practitioner must take control quickly; there is no time for debate, action is required. The authoritarian approach ensures the team responds immediately to preserve the patient's life. In contrast, in a staff meeting discussing changes to SACT processes, using a purely authoritarian approach can leave team members feeling undervalued and disempowered. If suggestions or concerns are dismissed, engagement drops, morale suffers, and the implementation of changes may fail, regardless of the potential benefits.

Delegative Leadership

Delegative or laissez-faire leadership provides team members with significant autonomy, allowing them to make decisions independently. This approach can encourage highly skilled and experienced staff to thrive, promoting productivity and professional growth. For instance, when reviewing a patient's blood results before treatment, an experienced SACT practitioner may autonomously decide to defer treatment due to unsafe results, inform the relevant team members, make alternative arrangements, and reassure the patient. This form of leadership in this scenario demonstrates trust and empowerment. However, the delegative approach can be risky for newer or less experienced staff. Without guidance, they may feel unsupported, make unsafe decisions, or misalign with local policy, potentially affecting patient safety. Even experienced practitioners new to a team may encounter the same challenges if policies differ between organisations, which in most cases it does. In these situations, delegative leadership can lead to disengagement, low morale and lack of accountability.

Transactional Leadership

Transactional leadership is a task-focused approach that emphasises hierarchy, rules and accountability. It relies on clearly defined roles, expectations and procedures, with rewards and consequences linked to performance. In SACT services, this style ensures that protocols are followed to the letter, reducing errors and supporting patient safety. Like all leadership styles, transactional leadership has both strengths and limitations. For example, during a routine treatment administration, you have completed pre-treatment checks, reviewing toxicities confirms patient identity and verifies the prescription. By following policy and adhering to these structured steps, the patient is kept safe and the risk of errors is minimised. However, a strictly transactional approach can sometimes overlook the holistic elements of care. In this scenario, focusing solely on "ticking the boxes" may result in missing signs of patient anxiety, discomfort or a need for reassurance, potentially affecting their overall experience and quality of life. While transactional leadership is highly effective for maintaining safety, consistency and accountability, it requires balance with approaches that consider patient experience and well-being.

Transformational Leadership

Transformational leadership is about inspiring and motivating others, often described as an attitude of energy, enthusiasm and passion for the task at hand. It is collaborative, engaging patients or teams in creating shared goals and visions. In SACT, transformational leadership can improve team morale, job satisfaction and patient compliance.

For example, involving patients in treatment decisions fosters patient concordance, while engaging the team in service improvements encourages innovation and shared ownership. However, this style can be demanding for the leader. Constant enthusiasm requires resilience and self-awareness to prevent burnout. It may also be less effective with individuals who resist energetic approaches, creating frustration if the leader cannot adapt. In high-pressure SACT settings, where staff are overworked or teams face daily challenges, transformational leadership must be applied thoughtfully to avoid disengagement while still motivating those who respond well to it.

Compassionate Leadership

Compassionate leadership is considered a supportive approach to leading; it displays empathy and understanding, supporting both patients and colleagues. It is about being aware of the experiences and needs of others, actively listening and responding in a way that promotes trust and psychological safety. In the SACT setting, where patients experience anxiety and staff are working in emotionally demanding environments, this approach to leadership is essential. If you were caring for a patient who is visibly distressed prior to treatment, as a compassionate leader you would take the time to listen, provide reassurance and adapt your communication to meet the needs of the patient. Similarly, you may notice when a colleague is overwhelmed with a situation and you may offer support, guidance, or simply a place to talk without prejudice or judgment. This approach can strengthen relationships but also improve team morale and enhance the patient experience, contributing to that person-centred approach. However, compassionate leadership can present some challenges if not balanced with other leadership styles. Focusing on emotional support alone may cause difficulties when needing to address performance concerns or unsafe practice. For example, if someone is adopting compassionate leadership alone, they may avoid giving constructive feedback to a colleague who is struggling, which could impact team effectiveness or patient safety. In high-pressure environments like SACT environments, there is also a risk that constantly supporting others without setting boundaries can lead to emotional fatigue or burnout. Meaning, compassionate leadership is most effective when combined with clear expectations and accountability.

Teams

In SACT, care is never delivered by one person alone, it is the result of a team working together, often under pressure to achieve a shared goal. But what is truly meant by the word "team"? In its simplest form, a team is a group of people working together towards a common goal. In SACT, that goal is clear: it is to deliver safe, effective and person-centred cancer treatment. However, a team is more than just a group of people working in the same place. It involves shared responsibility, mutual respect and an understanding of each other's roles. Teams come in different sizes, meaning it may be limited to the people working within the SACT unit or ward. However, the SACT team can also stretch across multiple services, which include nurses, pharmacists, doctors, healthcare support workers, dieticians, occupational therapists, counsellors and administrative staff, who all contribute in different ways to the patient's journey. Teams are vital in SACT provision because of the complexity and risk associated with treatment.

No single healthcare professional holds all the knowledge required to deliver care safely and effectively, so we must utilise each other's skill sets to increase team effectiveness. For example, pharmacists ensure the accuracy and safety of SACT preparation, nurses assess patients and administer treatment, and counsellors provide support required based on the psychological impact of SACT. Without effective communication and coordination between these professionals, the risk of error increases significantly and the quality of person-centred coordinated care is negatively affected.

Beyond safety, teams also play a crucial role in managing workload and supporting one another. SACT environments can be fast-paced and emotionally demanding. Having a supportive team allows team members to share the responsibility, seek advice when needed and manage challenging situations more effectively together. This is particularly important during high-pressure scenarios, such as managing adverse reactions with unexpected changes in a patient's episode of care or condition. The way a team functions has a direct impact on patient care. A well-coordinated team ensures that patients are prepared appropriately for treatment, monitored effectively during administration and supported afterwards. This includes everything from ensuring informed consent is obtained (see Chapter 4), recognising early signs of toxicity (see Chapter 6) and provide reassurance when patients feel anxious (see Chapter 11). When teamwork is strong, care feels seamless to the patient. When it is not, gaps can appear, communication can break down and patient experience and safety can be compromised. Ultimately, effective teamworking in SACT is more than completing set tasks, it is about delivering coordinated care that meets the individual needs of each patient. Leadership plays a key role in enabling this, but every member of the team contributes to how well it functions.

Stop and Think

Reflect on your current SACT team. How do you contribute to effective teamwork and how does your team influence patient safety and experience?

Team Culture

Teamwork is about what we do together, whereas team culture is about how we do it. It shapes the way people communicate, make decisions, support one another and ultimately how care is delivered to patients. Team culture is based on the team's shared values and the behaviours and attitudes within a team. In SACT settings, this includes how openly team members communicate, how comfortable they feel raising concerns and how they respond to both routine care and high-pressure situations. In a positive team culture, there is mutual respect, psychological safety and a shared commitment to delivering high-quality care. Team members feel able to ask questions, seek support and challenge decisions when needed. This is particularly important in SACT, where treatments carry significant risk, or issues may arise, such as toxicity or adverse reactions (see Chapter 6 and 7). On the flip side, a toxic team culture can have serious consequences. Poor communication, lack of support, or fear of speaking up can lead to errors, missed concerns and reduced quality of care. For example, if a practitioner feels unable to question a prescription or escalate concerns about a patient's condition, patient safety may be

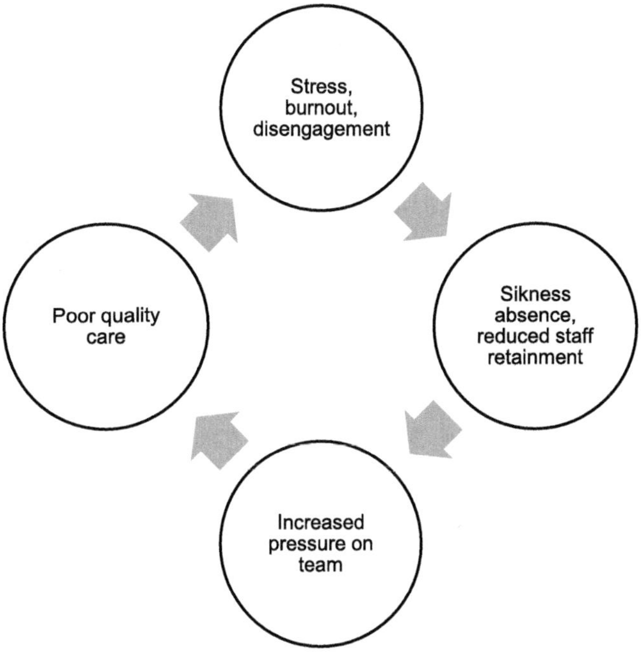

Figure 12.2 Image of the cycle of impact of a toxic culture on patient care

compromised. A toxic culture can also affect staff well-being, leading to stress, burnout, disengagement, sickness and absence, and a high level of staff turnover, which further impacts team performance based on morale and increased burden, leading to a negative impact on the continuity and quality of care. This is a self-perpetuating cycle, which can be seen in Figure 12.2.

A key element of a strong team culture is having a shared vision and common goals. In SACT, this often centres on delivering safe, effective and person-centred care. When teams are aligned in this way, decision-making becomes more consistent and individuals understand how their role contributes to the wider patient journey. It also helps prioritise what matters most, especially in busy or pressurised environments, as it closely links to person-centred care. When a team shares the same goal of focusing on the patient's needs, preferences and experiences, care becomes more coordinated and meaningful. Patients are more likely to feel informed, supported and involved in their treatment. In contrast, where team goals are unclear or inconsistent, care can become fragmented, with patients receiving mixed messages or feeling overlooked. Leadership plays a critical role in shaping and sustaining team culture. Leaders influence how teams communicate, how safe individuals feel to speak up, and how shared goals are understood and maintained. In SACT settings, effective leadership helps create an environment where staff feel supported to deliver safe care, reflect on practice, and continuously improve. More importantly, as mentioned earlier, leadership is not limited to those in senior roles, every member of the team contributes to culture through their behaviours, interactions and willingness to support others and therefore has the power to help shape the culture within the team.

Stop and Think

How do you support a positive team culture?

Summary

In summary, we have explored the evolution of leadership theories and considered how these can be applied in practice. We have examined different leadership styles, recognising that effective leaders need to adapt their approach according to the situation, context and team or patient needs. In addition, we have also explored how strong leadership can promote effective teamwork and how working collaboratively towards a shared goal, whether in a small or extended team, supports the delivery of high-quality, coordinated patient-centred care.

References

Bass, B.M. and Avolio, B.J. (1994) *Improving organizational effectiveness through transformational leadership*. Thousand Oaks: Sage.

Carlyle, T. (1974) *On heroes, hero-worship and the heroic in history*. Oxford University Press, Oxford.

Francis, R. (2013) *Report of the Mid Staffordshire NHS Foundation Trust Public Inquiry*. London: The Stationery Office.

Northouse, P.G. (2022). *Leadership: Theory and practice*. 9th edition. London: Sage.

Nursing and Midwifery Council (2018) *Future nurse: Standards of proficiency for registered nurses*. London: NMC.

Sinek, S. (2014) *Leaders eat last: Why some teams pull together and others don't*. New York: Portfolio/Penguin.

West, M., Eckert, R., Collins, B. and Chowla, R. (2017) *Caring to change: How compassionate leadership can stimulate innovation in health care*. London: The King's Fund. Accessed [online] 04 March 2026 via: https://assets.kingsfund.org.uk/f/256914/x/0b76247d02/caring_to_change_2017.pdf

Index

Note: Tables are indicated by **bold**.

For Product Safety Concerns and Information please contact our EU representative GPSR@taylorandfrancis.com Taylor & Francis Verlag GmbH, Kaufingerstraße 24, 80331 München, Germany

Batch number: 10726306

Printed by Printforce, the Netherlands